THE FIRST BOOK OF
Chakras

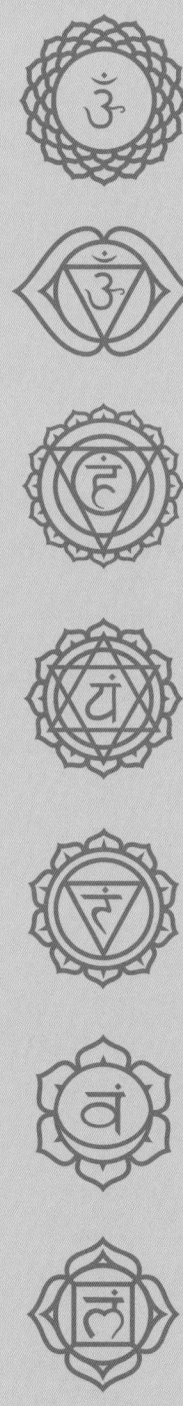

THE FIRST BOOK OF
Chakras

A Beginner's Guide to Harnessing Your Chakras
and Living a More Balanced Life

Jessica Allen

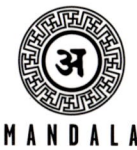

MANDALA

SAN RAFAEL LOS ANGELES LONDON

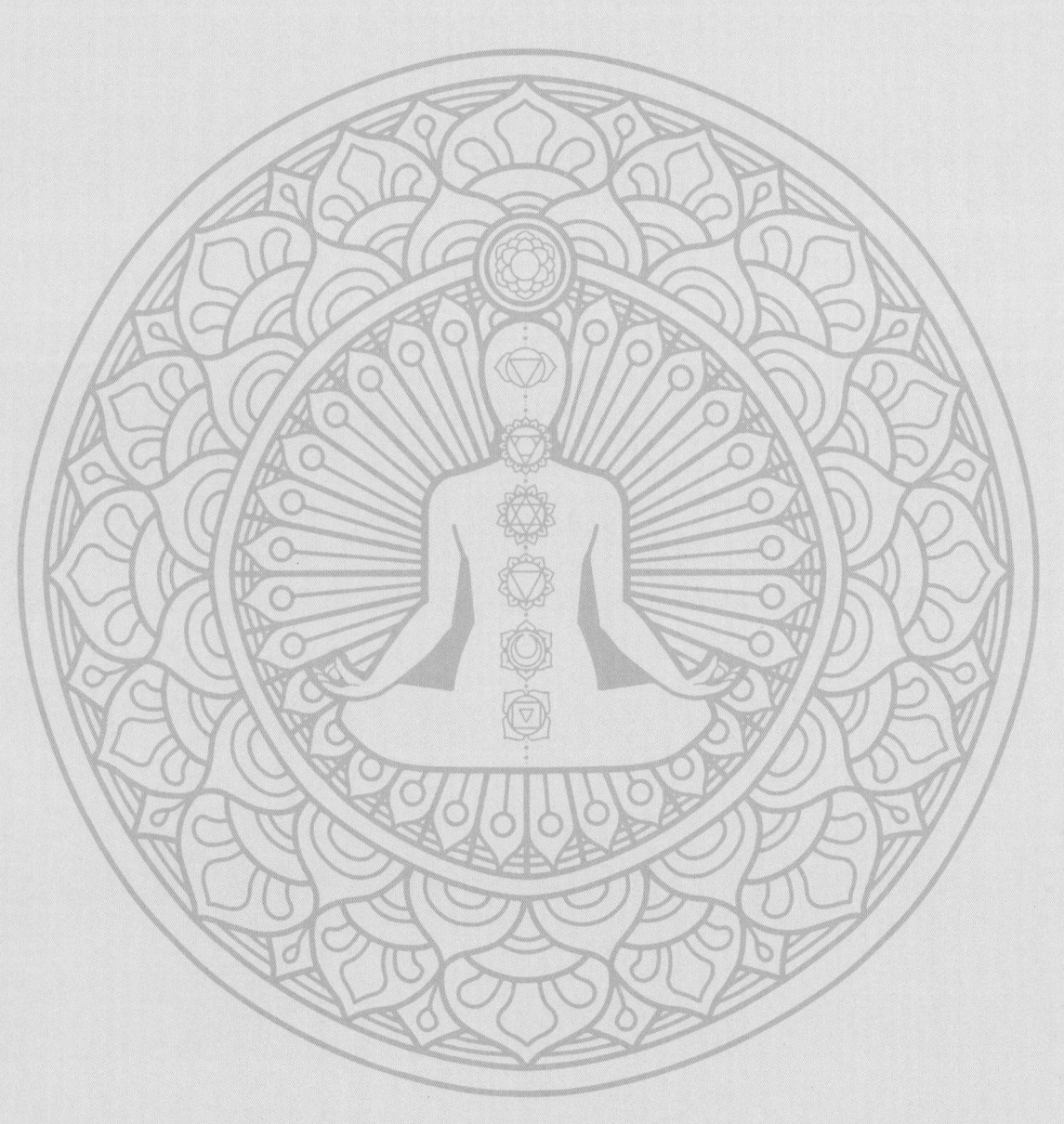

To Garrett, model of balance and more

Contents

INTRODUCTION — 09

The Seven Major Chakras

- Root Chakra — 25
- Sacral Chakra — 35
- Solar Plexus Chakra — 45
- Heart Chakra — 55
- Throat Chakra — 67
- Third Eye Chakra — 79
- Crown Chakra — 91

COMMON AILMENTS & AFFILIATED CHAKRAS — 103

FINAL THOUGHTS — 109

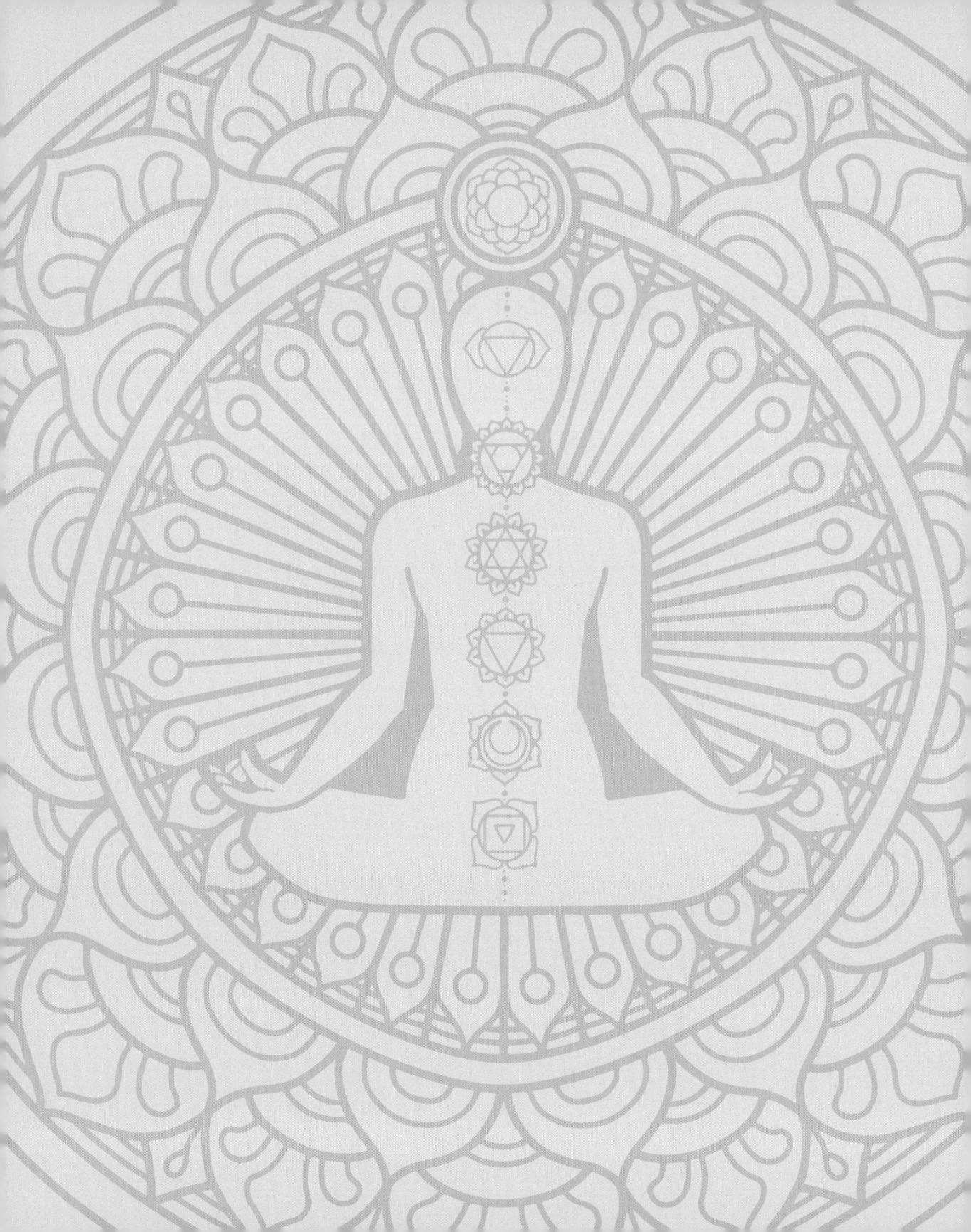

INTRODUCTION

As we live our lives, we create energetic effects. When we hug someone, for example, our molecules mix with their molecules. Indeed, our DNA hovers in the air around us and lingers when we leave the room. If we smile at a stranger, we inject positive energy into their day, which might later encourage that person to wave a car ahead of them in traffic, which could help that driver arrive home in a good mood, eager to help their kid with homework—and so on. Of course, the opposite holds as when negativity festers and intensifies. Either way, we are always giving off and receiving energy, in an infinite series of interconnections.

WHAT ARE CHAKRAS?

Chakras are invisible centers of spiritual and physical energy within the body. Much like molecules or good vibes, this energy affects how we relate to the world as well as how the world relates to us. Concentrating on the health of our chakra system can boost our well-being and be an important part of a holistic wellness practice—one of many tools we have to keep us healthy, strong, loving, confident, and capable of both fulfilling our goals and accessing a better version of ourselves.

Chakra is a Sanskrit word meaning *wheel* or *disk*. The concept of chakras was first described in the Indus Valley around 1500 BCE, as part of the ancient religious Hindu texts known as the Vedas. However, the idea of energy moving through and around the physical body likely took root long before, as people sought ways of understanding and describing the relationship between the seen and unseen world.

INTRODUCTION

> ## Chakra Pronunciation ॐ
> The word *chakra* is pronounced with a hard *ch*, as in *cheddar*, not the *sh* of *shark*.

Like Hinduism, Buddhism also uses the concept of chakras to describe spiritual energy moving in and around us. You might have heard about chakras during yoga class. Many yoga teachers and holistic practitioners will refer to *prana*, or centers, where energy gathers or intensifies in the body. If these centers become unbalanced, blocked, or drained, we may experience an array of physical, mental, and emotional ailments. We won't feel right.

Although the chakra system developed as part of Eastern spiritual traditions, scientists have begun to uncover correspondences between chakras and neural networks and other physiological components within the body. Although the approach might be different, you could say the ultimate goal is the same: to access and explore the connections between mind and body, the physical and metaphysical, and what we know and what we sense.

Everyday stressors can throw off the chakra system, as can larger issues like disease and trauma. Whether you're new to wellness work, or have an established self-care practice, focusing on your chakras can help you address various afflictions and improve your health.

What Do Chakras Do?

Chakras connect to and influence various aspects of our lives, including our bodily organs, feelings and moods, and self-identity.

When using the word *chakra*, the reference is to one of the seven major chakras, which can be categorized into three groups. Generally the three lower chakras concern earthly matters and physical health. The three upper chakras deal with spiritual matters. The heart chakra acts as a bridge between the two groups.

INTRODUCTION

SEVEN MAJOR CHAKRAS			
LOWER CHAKRAS			BROAD CONCERNS
Root Chakra	Sacral Chakra	Solar Plexus Chakra	Earthly matters, physical health
BRIDGE			
Heart Chakra			Connects lower and upper chakras
UPPER CHAKRAS			
Throat Chakra	Third Eye Chakra	Crown Chakra	Spiritual matters

Where Are the Chakras?

The seven major chakras are located at different points along the body, from the base of the spine to the top of the head. Each chakra, or energy center, has an associated Sanskrit name and color, among other connections we'll explore throughout this book. Imagining a particular color at a particular location along the body is a simple visualization exercise that can help you start to access your chakras, if you're new to this type of exploration.

SEVEN MAJOR CHAKRAS				
CHAKRA	SANSKRIT NAME	LOCATION	KEY ASSOCIATIONS	COLOR
Root	Muladhara	Base of the spine	Basic needs, safety, security	Red
Sacral	Svadhish-thana	2 inches (5 cm) below the belly button	Creativity, pleasure, sensuality	Orange

INTRODUCTION

Solar Plexus	Manipura	Middle of the torso between the belly button and breastbone	Confidence, drive, self-worth	Yellow
Heart	Anahata	Center of the chest	Compassion, empathy, love	Green
Throat	Vishuddha	Base of the throat	Authenticity, communication, truth	Blue
Third Eye	Ajna	Between the eyebrows	Imagination, inner wisdom, intuition	Indigo
Crown	Sahasrara	Top of the head	Connection, enlightenment, sense of purpose	Violet, white

While *The First Book of Chakras* focuses on the seven major chakras, many people believe the body contains upward of 88,000 chakras. Among those are the so-called minor chakras, which support the major chakras and contribute to equilibrium and stability in the body. Once you are familiar with the major chakras, you may wish to explore the minor chakras, delving into other resources as appropriate.

Palm Chakra

Although discussing the minor chakras is beyond the scope of this book, it's worth mentioning the palm chakra, or the energy center that influences loving touches, acts of service, and the giving of gifts, among other things. To activate your palm chakra, rub your hands together vigorously for 10–15 seconds. The heat and energy you feel are a sign of its activation. Place your warmed hands anywhere on your body that feels knotty or tense, or hold your hands in front of you and imagine a wheel of light spinning there.

Why Your Chakras Matter

Tending to your chakras can help you reduce stress, combat negativity, and increase well-being. This type of wellness work also improves self-awareness, which can benefit your relationships and interactions with others. Feeling more capable and confident in the world will help you identify and achieve your goals. More broadly, any healing work is almost always good, beneficial work.

Balanced and Unbalanced Chakras

When people talk about chakras, they might use words like *blocked*, *aligned*, *open*, and *balanced* to describe how the chakra is functioning. I prefer the terms *balanced* and *unbalanced*.

Consider a lotus flower, often used to symbolize the chakras. In this analogy, a balanced chakra is like an open flower, with petals spread and healthy, radiating and accepting. A balanced chakra allows energy to move easily and effortlessly in and around locations in the body, conferring a multitude of positive effects. An unbalanced chakra, in contrast, has its petals folded in protectively, as if closed off from everything. An unbalanced chakra might be overactive, spinning too quickly, or underactive, not spinning well enough. Only you will know when you're feeling off and in what ways. However, signs that your chakra system could be dysregulated include feeling isolated and separated from others, including a sense of dislocation from yourself. You might have low or no energy, or be apathetic and aimless.

Unlike a fever or fit of crying, a chakra that needs adjustment won't necessarily have an outward or easily identifiable symptom. Rather, you need to look within as well as consider myriad possible causes. Be careful about painting with a broad chakra brush or trying to diagnose different conditions. Use your explorations of your chakras as an opportunity to practice holistic healing—and reach out to a licensed medical professional for guidance when necessary.

INTRODUCTION

Giving your chakras care and consideration via visualizations, breathwork, or affirmations can provide immediate relief—all the more reason to carry your chakra affirmation cards, included with this book, with you as you go about the world, as they suggest simple everyday activities to boost each chakra. As in exercise, when an instructor asks you to think about your core while doing crunches, you can employ the mind-body connection to help align and adjust your chakras. Remember that simply sending your energy to a chakra can confer terrific benefits.

HOW TO USE THIS BOOK

The overarching goal of this book is to educate and empower you to explore your chakras while offering a range of techniques that might be familiar to you—such as meditation, yoga poses and stretches, and breathwork—to do so.

Each chakra chapter offers activities you can incorporate easily into your life or that you may currently be doing. You know yourself best so lean in to this book's modular sections with a sense of adventure and openness.

The book moves progressively up the body, from the root chakra to the crown chakra. Take as much time as you need to explore the different methods, practices, and recommendations. If you'd rather start somewhere else, turn to whatever chakra speaks to you right now, or explore the chakra related to a mindset you're hoping to incorporate more fully into your life (see pages 21-22). Listen to your body.

- In addition to the seven previously mentioned cards included with this book, you'll also find a wall chart showing the approximate locations of the seven major chakras in the body and a chakra healing bracelet.

- The cards are small enough to fit into a purse or a pocket so you can access your practice and balance your chakras pretty much anywhere.

- You may find it helpful to hang the chart in a special place dedicated to your spiritual practice, such as near an altar, or you may wish to bring it out when you're doing chakra-focused work.

- Simply wearing your bracelet can help balance your chakras, but if you wish to receive energy, wear it on your left wrist, and if you wish to put energy into the world, wear it on your right wrist. You can meditate on your bracelet and use it to receive awareness from and send awareness to each chakra by concentrating your attention there.

Wearing Your Chakra Healing Bracelet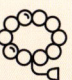

Before you put on your bracelet, set an intention. Which chakra or area of your life requires focus and care? It's totally fine if your intention is a broad desire to explore your chakras. The point, though, is to start to connect to your chakras.

Excited as you may be to dive into using these materials, I recommend reading a chapter or two first to get a feel for which exercises or activities seem most appropriate and doable for you. Perhaps you'll find a suggestion that dovetails with current wellness work. Then, you can begin making chakra-related tweaks as appropriate.

GETTING STARTED

To start exploring your chakras, begin with an open mind and a willingness to treat yourself with grace. You might not experience what you want to experience right away, or you might find some activities stirring up surprising sensations. Above all, be patient with yourself—and take a few minutes to appreciate your efforts to enhance well-being and deepen your understanding of the world through chakras.

A ritual tells your body and your mind that it's time to begin, much like your dog begins wagging her tail when you grab a leash. Your chakra ritual could be to play a certain song or put on a special outfit, or you could sit in a dedicated part of your space. You could wear your bracelet or reflect on your chart. Distractions happen, of course, but it can be helpful to use a ritual or gesture to clear your mind and set the right mood before beginning your work.

Keeping a notebook nearby allows you to capture any thoughts or feelings immediately that arise while undertaking your chakra work. Throughout the chakra chapters, there are journal prompts. You may wish to return to these prompts, especially as you start to see the benefits and effects of your efforts.

Unsure Where to Start?

If you're unsure about where to start, consider starting with the root chakra. Balancing this chakra can provide significant benefits as it encompasses basic needs, such as safety, shelter, and security. Without meeting these fundamental needs, concentrating on anything else will be almost impossible.

How to Get Started with Visualization Meditation

During a visualization meditation, we use our imagination to picture a certain image or person to achieve a particular end, such as relaxing, setting a goal, or improving overall well-being. You may already have a meditation practice, in which case adding visualizations may come naturally. Or, this might be your first time exploring this technique. Visualization meditation can sometimes be easier or more accessible than other types of meditation because you're giving your mind something specific to think about.

Among the most common ways of accessing the chakras is to visualize spinning wheels at different locations along the body. But other types of visualizations work, including envisioning the colors related to the chakras. When visualizing colors, try to imagine the platonic ideal of that color—its truest, shiniest, brightest, loveliest form. That said, avoid getting fixated on shade or tint. There are a million blues, of course, so picture the color that comes up for you when you hear "blue."

When (not if!) your mind wanders during visualization or other forms of meditation, gently bring your focus back. Try not to become fixated on what else you're thinking about, or annoyed that you lost focus. Instead, let the image or thought pop up, then float away, like a cloud drifting across the sky. Random thoughts are normal, especially if you're just starting with meditation. The key is to acknowledge those thoughts without getting emotionally caught up in or distracted by them.

How to Collect and Care for Crystals

Along with being lovely to look at, crystals can help us access the chakras. You can incorporate crystals into your wellness work by placing them around your home, holding them during meditation or while writing in your journal, putting them on your body, or wearing them as jewelry. Another effective means of using crystals is to keep one in your hand while reciting your affirmations.

Different crystals require different types of care. Not all crystals can be submerged in water, for example, so pay attention to the instructions you receive when acquiring your crystals. You might find that certain crystals benefit from being charged by sunlight or moonlight, or submerged in sea salt. Perhaps the most important consideration for working with crystals is to set aside your skepticism. Believing in crystals' benefits goes a long way toward manifesting those benefits.

Clear Quartz

Many wellness experts consider clear quartz to be a "master healer." It's thought to have cleansing properties, removing negative energy and embodying positivity. This powerful, purifying crystal can help balance all your chakras, so investing in one may add to your chakra practice.

How to Use Essential Oils

Essential oils can benefit the chakra system. To use, add a few drops to your shower or bath, or dab some on your body (after mixing with a carrier oil like coconut or olive oil). Another common way to work with essential oils is to inhale them, directly or through an aromatherapy diffuser.

Before incorporating any essential oils into your wellness practice, do the research and speak with a medical professional as necessary. If you're planning to apply essential oils directly to the skin, perform a patch test first to identify any sensitivities, prevent rashes, and avoid irritation. On their own, essential oils can be powerful to the point of overwhelming—a few drops should be enough to get the full benefits.

Lavender Oil

Lavender oil is thought to aid all the chakras and has been shown to combat insomnia, depression, and anxiety. Mix a few drops of lavender oil with a few drops of carrier oil, then massage on your temples to help with headaches or to help yourself relax into sleep.

How to Use Affirmations and Mantras

Affirmations are simple statements that can boost your self-confidence, combat negative thoughts, and give you courage and energy. To be effective, your affirmation should be positive, uplifting, and specific. Saying your affirmation out loud helps convince your brain to treat the statement as fact.

Each chapter includes affirmations related to each chakra, as do the chakra cards that accompany this book. If my suggestions don't speak to you, feel free to come up with your own. Focus on a characteristic or trait you appreciate about yourself that relates to the chakra in question. Repeat your affirmations throughout the day as necessary, or set aside specific times, such as

INTRODUCTION

when you're getting ready in the morning or preparing to go to bed. For added benefits, try holding a crystal while repeating your affirmation.

You'll also find mantras connected to each chakra. Also known as *bija mantras* or *seed sounds*, these words can help you access your chakras. You can sit, stand, or lie in a comfortable position while chanting your mantra. You might also try closing your eyes and focusing on the associated chakra's location as you chant. Keep in mind, too, that chanting doesn't have to be a major production—you can repeat the sound quietly to yourself as you move about your day or while looking at your chakra cards.

How to Connect to Your Chakras

A balanced chakra feels different for everyone. Some people report a tingling sensation whereas others feel an energetic lift radiating from the chakra's location. Others feel better overall, riding a sense of calm and well-being that enables them to tackle or enjoy whatever life sends their way.

Of course, before you can balance your chakras, you need to connect with them. Try this "getting in touch" exercise as a first step. Remember, your goal at this point is to familiarize yourself with your chakras—thinking about and sending energy to your chakras will help you prepare for more focused work later in this book. Indeed, as noted, sometimes simply thinking about your chakras, visualizing their colors, and imaging what each chakra offers, can be enough to make the mind-body-chakra connection.

Full-Body Scan Chakra Visualization

Sometimes called the "rainbow meditation," this exercise can help you align your entire chakra system. You may find it helpful to visualize the colors as balls or wheels, or you may wish to imagine rays of light. What matters most is that you picture colors at the chakras—again, no need to stress about shades—and send your powerful, benevolent energy to the chakra system.

1. Find a quiet place to sit or lie down.
2. Take a few deep breaths as you close your eyes and relax.
3. Turn your attention inward and focus on your root chakra, at the base of your spine. Visualize the color red, providing safety and stability, and connecting you to the earth.
4. Move your focus up the body to the sacral chakra, 2 inches (5 cm) below your belly button. Visualize the color orange, filling you with creativity.
5. Move to the solar plexus chakra, between your belly button and breastbone, beneath your rib cage. Visualize the color yellow, infusing you with confidence.
6. Transition to the heart chakra, at the center of your chest. Visualize the color green, beaming out and surrounding you with love.
7. Continue up the body to the throat chakra, at the base of your throat. Visualize the color blue, helping you communicate and speak your truth.
8. Move to the third eye chakra at the center of your forehead, just above your eyebrows. Visualize the color indigo, giving your mind focus, clearing out baggage, and allowing wisdom and insight to pour in.
9. Transition to the crown chakra, on top of, or slightly above, your head. Visualize the color violet or white, expanding your consciousness. (Both colors are associated with this chakra so pick the one that feels right to you.)
10. Imagine the seven chakras in alignment. Visualize all seven colors shining and pulsating at the same rate.
11. Take a few more breaths, noting any sensations.
12. Return your awareness to the world around you. Gently move your fingers and toes, and open your eyes when you're ready.

How to Know When It's Working (And When to Take a Break)

It's very easy to figure out when some practices are working—you start to run a faster mile, for example, or you're able to make a soufflé that doesn't collapse. While progress in your chakra work may have less obvious markers, you will, no doubt, benefit from a consistent practice. Remember to allow yourself to feel and experience whatever it is you're feeling and experiencing. Holding back can set you back.

When connecting with a chakra, you may feel warm, or you may get especially emotional, intensely laughing or crying for a few minutes. You might feel a sense of peace or lightness. Almost certainly, you'll be better able to regulate your emotions day to day. Decisions will be easier. Your path and purpose will start to become clearer.

Remember, too, that some days are better than others. If a specific practice or sensation isn't available to you on a given day, let it go. Take a break and do something else. Frustration is normal. As always, be patient and kind to yourself.

CHAKRAS AND MINDSETS

Chakras affect different states of mind, like beliefs, emotions, and feelings. Use the following chart to guide your chakra practice, identifying and focusing on the chakra that's related to a feeling you're looking to develop or strengthen in your life.

CHAKRAS AND MINDSETS	
MINDSET	RELATED CHAKRA(S)
Awe	Crown Chakra
Communication	Throat Chakra

INTRODUCTION

Connectedness	Crown Chakra
Contentment	Crown Chakra
Courage	Solar Plexus Chakra
Creativity	Sacral Chakra, Throat Chakra
Curiosity	Third Eye Chakra
Empathy	Heart Chakra, Crown Chakra
Enlightenment	Crown Chakra
Joy	Sacral Chakra
Love	Heart Chakra
Patience	Root Chakra
Resilience	Solar Plexus Chakra
Security	Root Chakra
Self-confidence	Solar Plexus Chakra
Self-knowledge	Third Eye Chakra
Sense of purpose	Crown Chakra
Stability	Root Chakra
Tranquility	Sacral Chakra, Crown Chakra
Trust	Root Chakra, Third Eye Chakra
Understanding	Crown Chakra
Wholeness	Crown Chakra

Easy Fixes for When You're Feeling Off

First of all, it's okay if you don't know where to start when you're not feeling quite right. Forgive yourself and let go of any expectations. Then, find a quiet place to lie down, close your eyes, and do a body scan. Beginning at your toes, slowly scan up your body, pausing and noting where you feel any discomfort or knots. Pay attention to any sensations without judgment. Let your body tell you what it needs. When you're ready, open your eyes, refer to your chakra wall chart, and home in on the chakra closest to the body part that felt a little sticky or troublesome.

Other fixes when you're feeling off:

- **Relax in a way that's meaningful and safe for you.** Being anxious or making poor lifestyle choices, such as forgoing exercise or eating an unhealthy diet, can negatively affect our chakras. Take a nap, practice yoga, or try a breathwork exercise.

- **Trust your intuition.** If you find yourself drawn to a particular chakra, listen to those feelings and give it some care. Refer to whatever chakra chapter speaks to you in this moment.

- **Wear your chakra healing bracelet.** Simply putting it on can help you center your awareness on your chakras, thereby giving them a positive energy boost. For a more harmonious, relaxing effect, wear your bracelet on your left wrist. If you need to actively combat negative energy, wear your bracelet on the right wrist.

Ultimately, your chakra work belongs to you. It won't feel the same from day to day, and some days you might find certain techniques more beneficial than other days. As ever, give yourself grace.

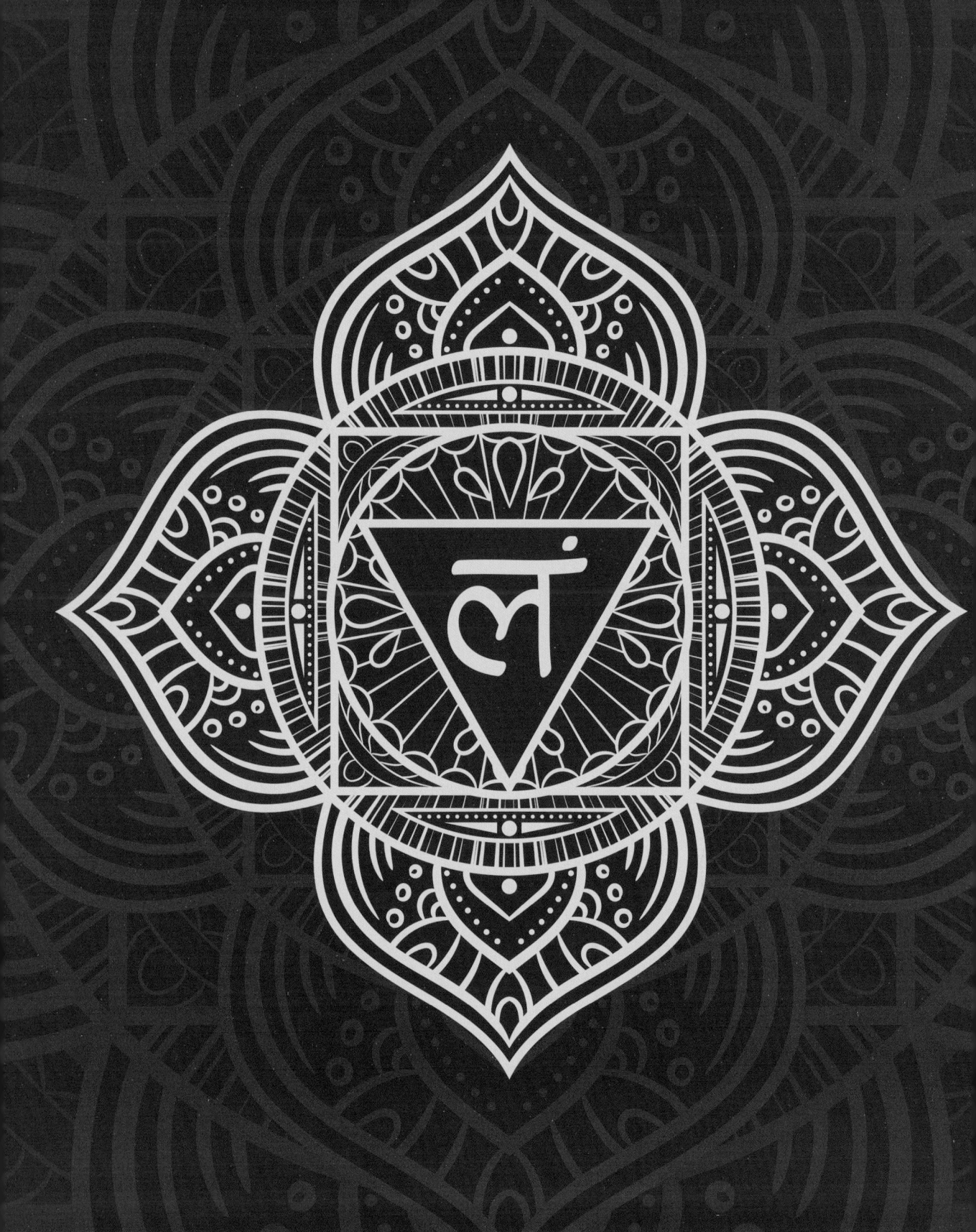

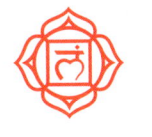

THE SEVEN MAJOR CHAKRAS

Root Chakra

A bear hug from a loved one. A healthy bank account. A pantry stocked with ingredients to make your famous chocolate chip cookies. A linen closet with a spare bottle of your favorite shampoo. A car parked in a driveway next to a house that's yours, plus a text chain that's been going on forever with your friends. Only you know what makes you feel most secure and safe.

Each of us intuitively understands the feeling of having our basic needs satisfied. As with many things, you know it when you feel it—and you're unsettled and upset when you don't. Such feelings of health and well-being are fundamental to our sense of self, crucial to our ability to thrive, and related to the root chakra.

Located at the base of the spine, the root chakra is associated with security, safety, and fundamental needs like food and shelter. Its Sanskrit name, *muladhara*, translates as "root" (*mula*) "support" (*adhara*). Among the feelings related to the root chakra are stability, survival, and stillness. A balanced root chakra helps you feel grounded. You're present. You're here. Everything's okay.

WHY BALANCING YOUR ROOT CHAKRA MATTERS

Balancing your root chakra gives you a firm foundation from which to operate. After all, this chakra is linked to such primal needs as having a roof over your head and knowing you have enough to eat. When those needs go unsatisfied, we scramble to rectify the situation as quickly as possible, often growing increasingly frazzled and frantic in the process.

Likewise, with our basic needs satisfied, we can turn to other facets of our lives, such as creativity and pleasure. We can act and react with patience. We confidently connect to others and the wider world around us. We feel at home, in all senses of the phrase.

The root chakra helps you stay present and grounded. It's affiliated with the body's waste control (excretory) system, including the colon, as well as the adrenal glands, spine, legs, and feet. Any of these body parts can get sore, blocked, or otherwise negatively affected if the root chakra is unbalanced.

What an Unbalanced Root Chakra Feels Like

When your root chakra is unbalanced, you may feel keyed up, as if your fight-or-flight response were firing nonstop. You may start to struggle with anxiety, confusion, fear, rejection, or constipation. You might be especially irritable or irrationally angry. Panicky and restless, your emotions seem to skitter away from you like a wayward child. Everything's off.

An overactive root chakra frequently leads to greediness, even hoarding. You want, you want more; you acquire, you acquire more. This tendency toward acquisitiveness may transfer to food, causing overindulgence and subsequent or related issues like bloating and heartburn.

We can also become too rooted as a result of an overactive root chakra, such that we grow stubborn, immobile, and resistant to change. Rather than going with the flow and living with ease, an unbalanced root chakra makes us feel insecure and agitated. We start to lose confidence.

Underactive, the root chakra often leads to a lack of motivation, an exhausted "Why bother?" attitude that—left unchecked—could tip into despair.

UNBALANCED ROOT CHAKRA	
PHYSICAL AILMENTS	MENTAL AND EMOTIONAL AILMENTS
Fatigue	Irritability
Overindulgence	Anxiety
Constipation	Insecurity
Leg or back pain	Immobility
Weight loss or gain	Disconnection

How to Balance Your Root Chakra

A balanced root chakra offers a sense of control, abundance, and protection. You have enough, and you are enough. You feel content, calm, and capable. Knowing that your basics are covered, you're free to focus on other things, like self-expression and relationships.

Visualizations and Meditations

Spin the wheel. Envision a red wheel near your coccyx (base of the spine), between your perineum and lower spine. Use your breath to make this wheel spin, or pace your breaths to its movement. As you watch the wheel turn, notice any sensations. Let yourself feel warm, safe, stable, secure, and present.

Meditate on the color red. Picture a beautiful red apple or luscious, ripe pomegranate. Visualizing joyful red things—like cherries, ladybugs, or a blooming red-leaf Japanese maple tree—can help you unlock your root chakra. Wearing an item of red clothing can help, too, as can wearing your chakra bracelet.

THE SEVEN MAJOR CHAKRAS | ROOT CHAKRA

Give yourself roots. Stand with your feet firmly planted on the ground. Close your eyes, and imagine roots extending from your base down your legs, through your feet, and into the earth beneath you. Although you can do this visualization anywhere, consider doing it near a tree or in a forest. Being near things with roots will help you strengthen your sense of your own.

Walk with intention. A walking meditation involves a level of concentration we don't normally bring to our everyday walks. Instead of rushing from place to place, walk slowly, articulating through the bones of your feet. Right now, during this meditation, all that matters is the walk itself, not the destination, not your to-do list. You can recite an affirmation, too, as you walk, or just concentrate on the sensation of moving across the earth.

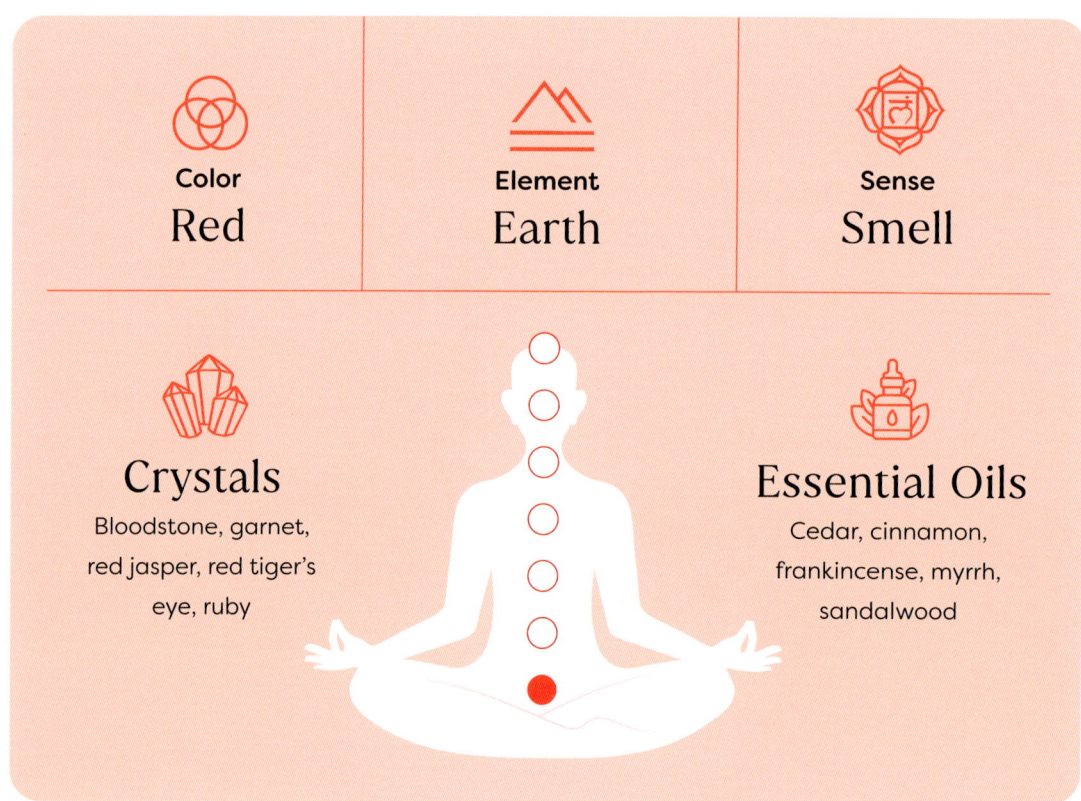

Color
Red

Element
Earth

Sense
Smell

Crystals
Bloodstone, garnet, red jasper, red tiger's eye, ruby

Essential Oils
Cedar, cinnamon, frankincense, myrrh, sandalwood

Food

Think earthy foods like root vegetables and whole grains, or foods that are the same (red) color as the root chakra, such as beets, red beans, raspberries, strawberries, or tomatoes. Nuts, tofu, and other protein-rich foods help you build muscle and feel strong, both of which contribute to overarching feelings of strength and stability.

Herbs and Spices

Black pepper, cayenne pepper, clove, ginger, sage

Yoga Poses and Stretches

Chair pose, malasana squat, mountain pose, tree pose, wide-legged forward fold

Breathwork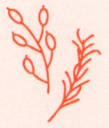

BELLY BREATHING

Belly breathing sends breath to the lower abdomen so you fill your body with breath, letting your lungs and diaphragm work together. Also called "diaphragmatic breathing," this type of breathing is used in many meditations—partly because it's incredibly simple, and partly because it's so effective at returning you to the fundamental act of breathing.

1. Lie flat, sit comfortably, or stand up straight.
2. Move your shoulders away from your ears. Relax.
3. Put one hand on your stomach and one hand on your chest.
4. Inhale through your nose, taking in as much air as is comfortable. Don't force it.

5. Pause briefly to let the air move around inside you. Feel your belly. Exhale by pursing your lips, as if you were sipping through a straw, for at least 4 seconds. Feel your belly contract. The hand on your chest shouldn't move.
6. Repeat a few more times.
7. Resume breathing normally.

THREE-PART BREATH

In this breathing technique, you concentrate on filling your belly, rib cage, and chest—aka the "three parts"—with air. Three-part breath helps deepen your inhales and exhales, which counteracts the shallow breathing that often occurs when we're nervous or stressed.

1. Lie flat or sit comfortably.
2. Move your shoulders away from your ears. Relax.
3. Put one hand on your stomach and one hand on your chest.
4. Inhale through your nose, sending breath first to your belly, then to your rib cage, and finally throughout your chest, up to your collarbones. Feel each part expand as it fills with breath.
5. Exhale through your nose by reversing the breath out of your chest, rib cage, and belly. Feel each part fall slightly as it empties.
6. Repeat a few more times, evening out your inhales and exhales.
7. Resume breathing normally.

Mantra Chant Sound

Lam (pronounced *luuummm*)

Affirmations

I am grounded. I am safe and secure.
I have enough. I am rooted.
I am at home in the world.

Flowers and Plants

Dandelion, hellebore, poppy, red currant, rose (red)

Acts of Service

Make a donation. Studies have shown that giving away money not only makes people feel happier but also makes them feel wealthier. In fact, a 2007 study using MRIs found that similar regions of the brain are activated when a person gives *or* receives money. In other words, giving away fifty dollars feels the same as receiving fifty dollars. Relatedly, when we give, we feel as though we have enough to give—this virtuous cycle increases feelings of satisfaction and gratification.

Plant a tree. If you have the space and the resources, planting a tree in your backyard will help bond you to your home and your neighborhood, ushering in a sensation of groundedness. If actually planting a tree isn't an option, plenty of organizations around the globe will do so on your behalf. Along with contributing to the beauty of our natural world, trees play a great role in mitigating the effects of climate change so the benefits of this act radiate beyond you to future generations.

Everyday Activities to Activate Your Root Chakra

Take off your shoes. Touching the earth with your toes can help you feel more grounded—literally. This technique works whether you discretely slip off your shoes at the office, or go outside and wander barefoot in the grass. Wiggle, stretch, shuffle, tiptoe, think about the earth's gravitational pull. How you touch the earth is up to you.

Care for plants. Gardening can benefit your root chakra by putting you in direct contact with things that grow in the earth. From root to root, for sure. Indoors, plants clean and purify the air, but greenery also fosters feelings of homeyness. Plants freshen our spaces as well as our lungs. Having plants nearby has been shown to boost creativity, and your sacral and throat chakras will benefit as well.

Dance. Dancing helps with balance, coordination, mobility, and stability. It lowers blood pressure, can improve memory, and has been shown to boost problem-solving abilities and other cognitive functions. Dancing is among the oldest of human art forms, joining us to the deep past. And, of course, dancing feels good. As you dance, focus on moving your feet, legs, and hips. Let the movement connect you to your root chakra.

Self-Care Rituals for Your Root Chakra

Declutter. While stocking up on various items often leads to feelings of contentment, having too much stuff can be problematic. We may feel overwhelmed and unable or unwilling to be tidy. Decluttering enables us to see—and love—what we have. We can take better care of our things because we don't possess an excess of them.

Keep a gratitude journal. Much like decluttering, keeping a gratitude journal fosters feelings of abundance and appreciation. Both activities encourage you to appreciate what you have right now, not what you want in the future. You can journal about material possessions, list what you like about your house, or give thanks for the people in your life. Another option is to focus on your body, from the breath that fills your lungs to the feet that take you where you want to go to the eyes that let you read these words.

Practice aromatherapy. While working with essential oils confers big benefits to all your chakras and enhances your overall sense of well-being, aromatherapy has special benefits for your root chakra: The root chakra is closely associated with our sense of smell. Massaging scented oil onto your body or setting up a diffuser is a low-key way to switch on the root chakra.

THE SEVEN MAJOR CHAKRAS | ROOT CHAKRA

Journal Prompts

- *When and where do you feel safest?*
- *What does the word security mean to you?*
- *As a child, what was your favorite smell?*
- *Draw or describe your ideal tree.*
- *What makes you feel organized and prepared to tackle the day's challenges?*
- *Why does balancing your root chakra matter to you at this moment?*

ROOT CHAKRA AT A GLANCE	
SANSKRIT NAME	Muladhara (moo-lahd-har-ah)
SYMBOL	Lotus flower with four petals
LOCATION	Base of the spine
THIS CHAKRA IS CONNECTED TO	Basic needs, safety, security, survival
COLOR	Red
CRYSTALS	Bloodstone, garnet, red jasper, red tiger's eye, ruby
ELEMENT	Earth
MANTRA	Lam
"I FEEL" AFFIRMATION	I feel safe and grounded
ANIMAL	Elephant
BENEFITS OF BALANCING THIS CHAKRA	Able to focus on other chakras and concerns, groundedness, satiety, sense of safety and security, stability
WHEN UNBALANCED	Anxiety, fear, insecurity, overindulgence, stubbornness

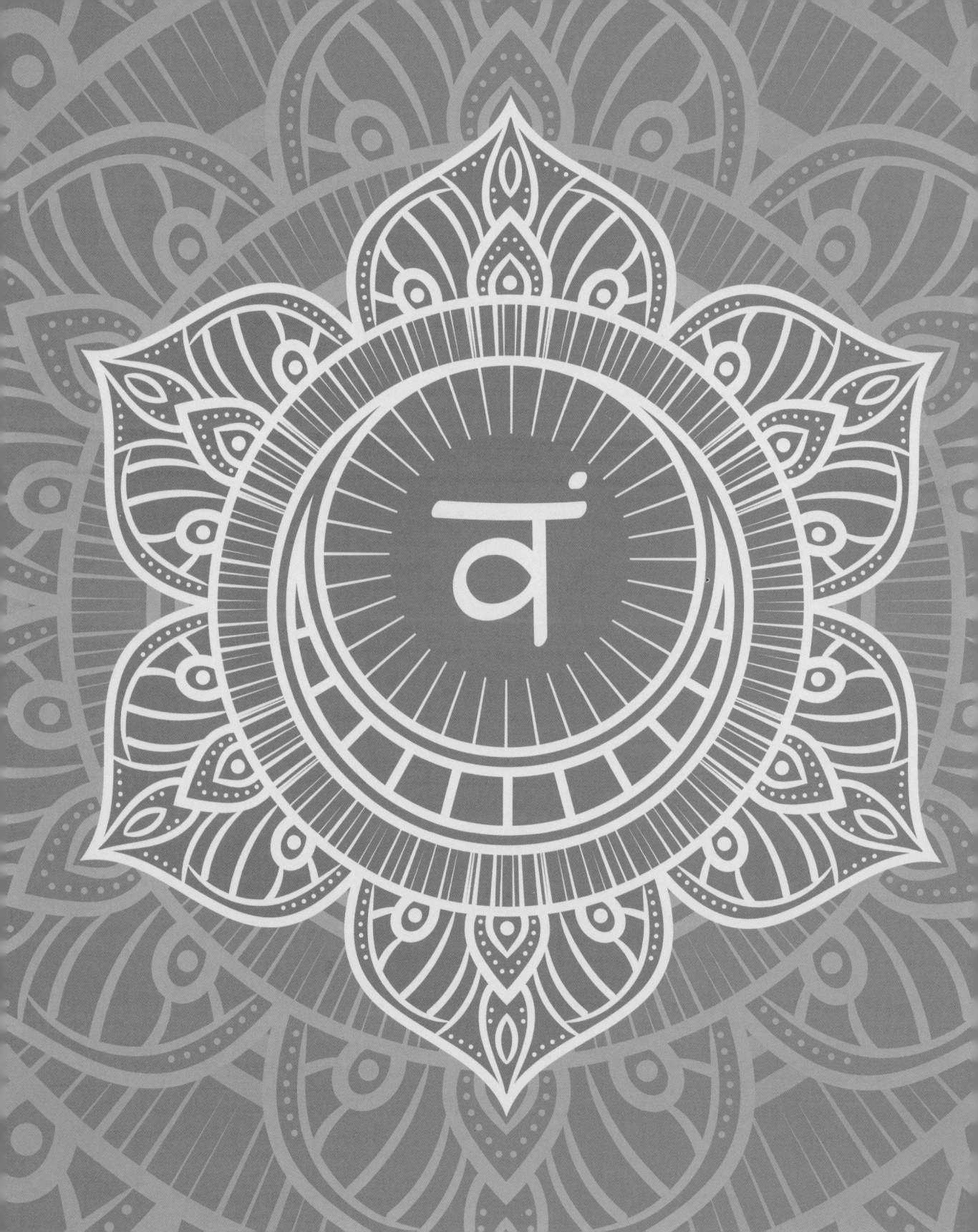

Sacral Chakra

In 2024, researchers uncovered a strong association between the color orange and happiness, with participants in one study identifying more words on an orange background with joy than words on a blue background. As a color, orange typically connotes optimism, warmth, enthusiasm, creativity, and excitement—and it's affiliated with the sacral chakra.

Located about 2 inches (5 cm) below the belly button, the sacral chakra encompasses our ability to feel pleasure in a variety of forms. It also relates to whether we can infuse our lives with joy, sweetness, and cheer; pursue creative endeavors; and appropriately regulate our emotions. You might say the sacral chakra is the happy chakra.

The sacral chakra is called *svadhishthana* in Sanskrit, often translated to "where you are established" or "where your being is found." These translations demonstrate the element of intimacy inherent in this chakra. After all, the sacral chakra is located near the genitals and can influence sexuality.

Creativity is also deeply personal. Bringing our imaginative creations into the world requires a considerable level of vulnerability, including a willingness to expose a unique part of ourselves. Ditto with emotions, some of which we might prefer to keep hidden. Yet being open and revealing these parts of us can lead to a profound feeling of completeness.

WHY BALANCING YOUR SACRAL CHAKRA MATTERS

A balanced sacral chakra gives you inspiration as well as the energy to put that creativity into action. You'll find more pleasure in daily life, from the froth on a latte to watching a flock of birds take off in flight, and you'll be more in touch with your senses. The number of positive interactions you have in a day will, no doubt, increase. "Laugh, and the world laughs with you" goes a nineteenth-century poem. Balance your sacral chakra, and the world will seem eager to receive what you have to offer.

In terms of what this bequeathing might look like, try to recall a time when you were in the flow—that is, when you were so consumed by a task that you didn't notice the passing of time. Basketball players might get in the flow when they practice layups, sculptors when they carve a new bust. Regardless of your endeavors, when your sacral chakra is blocked, you're unable to access this creative happy place. However, when balanced, your sacral chakra encourages you to share or seek out what you want to make, what you want to experience, and what you need to feel satisfied.

What an Unbalanced Sacral Chakra Feels Like

An unbalanced sacral chakra impedes us from experiencing life's joys. A food that used to taste delicious starts to taste like wet cardboard—all texture, no flavor. An activity that once delighted us leaves us unmoved, unstimulated, and unenthusiastic. It's as if someone turned our kaleidoscopic technicolor world into monochromatic shades of black, white, and gray.

When the sacral chakra is misaligned, we have trouble bonding with others. We retreat, shying away from fun as well as family and friends. Consequently, this lack of connection can lead to loneliness and isolation. When the sacral chakra is overfiring, our imagination might leap into hyperdrive. We might be brimming with ideas but unable to follow through.

In addition to creativity and pleasure, the sacral chakra helps regulate our emotions. As a result, when the sacral chakra is off, our emotions are also off—we might ping from one extreme to the other or have a tough time modulating. Indeed, we may overreact or react inappropriately. We might make up stories to justify our feelings, rather than relying on objective facts, getting creative with reality in a nonproductive way.

UNBALANCED SACRAL CHAKRA	
PHYSICAL AILMENTS	MENTAL AND EMOTIONAL AILMENTS
Urinary problems	Loneliness
Low libido	Mood swings
Sciatica	Indifference
Stiffness	Jealousy
Exhaustion	Lack of creativity

How to Balance Your Sacral Chakra

A balanced sacral chakra enables you to feel playful, cheerful, and joyful. You invite and experience pleasure. An effervescent sunniness infuses both your attitude and your life. You're open to countless possibilities—and full of the enthusiasm needed to make those possibilities come to fruition.

Visualizations and Meditations

Spin the wheel. Envision an orange wheel at your hips and lower abdomen. Use your breath to make this wheel spin, or pace your breaths to its movement. As you watch the wheel turn, notice any sensations. Let yourself feel sunny, upbeat, lively, and cheery.

Meditate on the color orange. Picture a juicy peach at the height of summer or a bunch of carrots, long and lean. Visualizing joyful orange things—like mandarins, pumpkins, goldfish, or a frolicsome orange cat—can help you unlock your sacral chakra. Wearing an item of orange clothing can help, too, as can wearing your chakra bracelet.

THE SEVEN MAJOR CHAKRAS | SACRAL CHAKRA

Watch the water. If you live near a river or an ocean, spend some time quietly contemplating its ebbs, flows, ripples, and swells. Let your eyes soften, maybe close. But you don't need to physically be near water to participate in this visualization—just imagine a body of water. Either way, the water's gentle movement can help your emotions settle and loosen any blockages related to your sacral chakra.

Eat a raisin. Fewer than 15 minutes of mindfulness meditation has been shown to boost creativity. An easy mindfulness meditation is to eat a raisin, pretending as though you've never encountered such a thing before. Focus on its size, shape, texture, and taste. What does it feel like? Explore its contours, stretching and smoothing, pushing and pulling. Play with it. Above all, devote your attention to truly noticing the raisin. Not a fan of raisins? Pick another familiar food, then render it unfamiliar and start to see it anew.

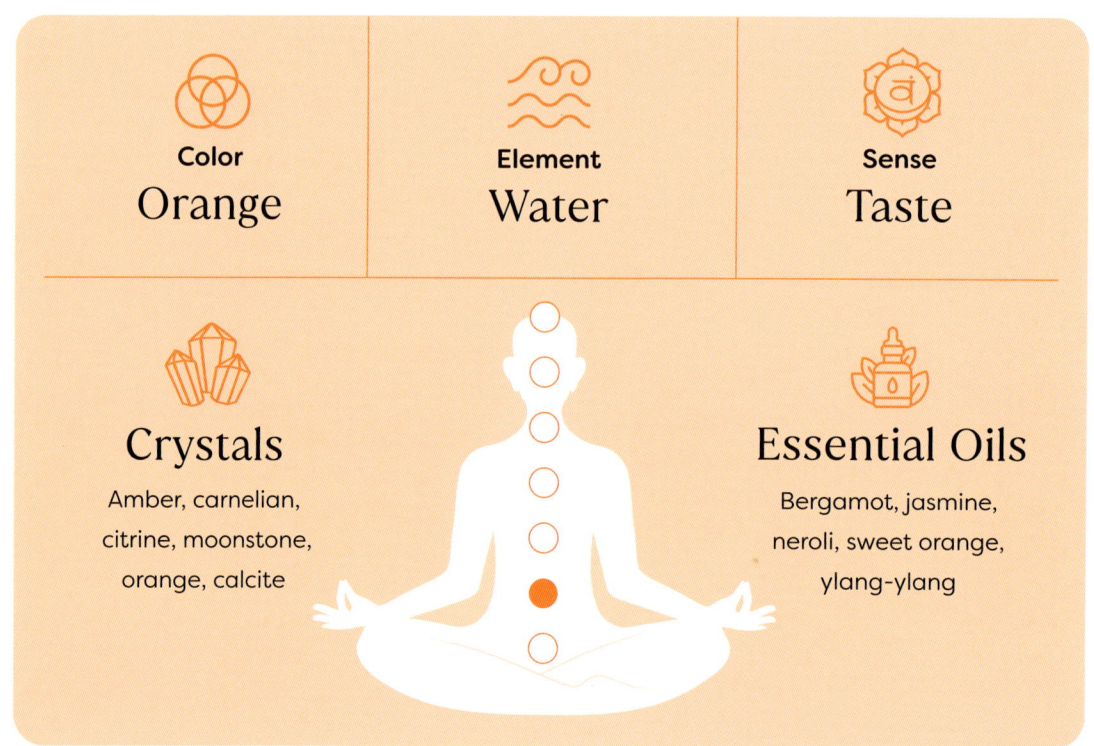

Color	Element	Sense
Orange	Water	Taste

Crystals
Amber, carnelian, citrine, moonstone, orange, calcite

Essential Oils
Bergamot, jasmine, neroli, sweet orange, ylang-ylang

THE SEVEN MAJOR CHAKRAS | SACRAL CHAKRA

Food

Aid your sacral chakra by staying hydrated with broths, soups, juices, and smoothies. Load up on bright, tropical flavors, like mango and papaya, which have the additional benefit of being orange. For an easy, filling soup, blend sautéed onion and roasted butternut squash with vegetable broth or a milk of your choosing.

Herbs and Spices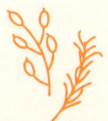

Cardamom, chamomile, hibiscus, orange mint, vanilla

Yoga Poses and Stretches

Butterfly pose, goddess pose, happy baby, pigeon pose, seated forward bend

Breathwork

ALTERNATE NOSTRIL BREATHING

As the name suggests, this breathwork practice involves breathing in and out through opposite nostrils, rather than both nostrils at the same time. While alternate nostril breathing can lead to a sense of calm, it can also help energize and inspire us, two mindsets that are wonderful for the sacral chakra.

1. Sit comfortably.
2. Move your shoulders away from your ears. Relax.
3. Hold your hand in front of your nose. Using a thumb or finger, gently close one nostril.
4. Inhale through the open nostril, then close it with a thumb or finger. Both nostrils are now closed.

THE SEVEN MAJOR CHAKRAS | SACRAL CHAKRA

5. Open the opposite nostril and exhale through it.
6. Inhale through that open nostril, then close it. Both nostrils are now closed.
7. Open the opposite nostril and exhale through it.
8. Repeat a few more times, making sure you have an equal number of inhales and exhales from each nostril.
9. Resume breathing normally.

HO-HO-HA-HA-HA

In laughter yoga, people complete a series of movements designed to elicit laughter and a sense of happiness. Borrow a warm-up chant known as Ho-Ho-Ha-Ha-Ha from this type of yoga practice to access your sacral chakra and add some play to your life.

1. Sit or stand comfortably.
2. Move your shoulders away from your ears. Relax.
3. Begin chanting "ho ho ha ha."
4. Clap softly as you chant. Use your claps to keep the beat. Inhales will happen naturally.
5. Sway or stay still. Be quiet or get loud. Keep going for as long as it feels right.
6. Resume breathing normally.

Mantra Chant Sound

Vam (pronounced *vuuummm*)

Affirmations

I am full of joy.
Creativity flows through me.
I am in control of my emotions.
I give and receive pleasure.
I bring joy to the world.

Flowers and Plants

Bird of paradise, butterfly weed, marigold, tiger lily, tulip

Acts of Service

Make a homemade card or gift. Sometimes we get caught up in distorted definitions of words like *creative*. The truth is that anyone can be creative—you don't need an MFA to write a poem or to draw a picture. What you do need, however, is to give yourself permission to experiment, to explore, and to play. So, set aside an afternoon to make a gift for a loved one. The right person (anyone who genuinely cares about you) will appreciate the effort.

Compliment someone. Tell a friend you like their haircut; praise a stranger for their choice of outfit. A nice word can make a person's day, lift their spirits, and encourage them to carry that joy forward, perhaps to praise someone they encounter. You'll feel buoyed as well so it's worth overcoming any anxiety or awkwardness you might feel about doling out the admiration. Instead, remember that an authentic expression of praise lifts the mood of the giver *and* the giftee, thereby boosting the sacral chakra.

Everyday Activities to Activate Your Sacral Chakra

Drink a glass of water. We humans are watery creatures. In fact, our brains are more than 70 percent water. Not drinking enough water leads to headaches, decreased cognitive function, and irritability. So, basically, if you're dehydrated, you can't think right. Pausing and sipping water also lets you calibrate your emotions and choose the right reaction, which is especially handy during a stressful situation.

Play. If you have a pet, get on the floor and tussle. If you have a child in your life, take them to a playground and run around, or spend an afternoon drawing. Animals and kids have a magical ability to be in the present playful moment that adults—with their self-consciousness and long to-do lists—often lack. Don't worry about how you look or what you're making. Concentrate on doing a fun activity that allows you to lose yourself for a while.

Be spontaneous. Go left instead of right. Make breakfast for dinner. Wear plaid with stripes. As busy people, we likely organize our days to maximize productivity and minimize waste, especially when it comes to the basics, like always doing certain things in the same way. That makes sense, but it can also cause us to fall into ruts and miss opportunities for whimsy and creativity.

Self-Care Rituals for Your Sacral Chakra

Take a bath. Connect to your sacral chakra by taking a soothing bath. Add some essential oils, if you wish, or a scented bath bomb. Pleasantly submerging yourself in water can help you access your sacral chakra. Water flows, much like creativity and emotions. As you soak, think about how feelings come and go. When you're done with the bath, unplug the drain and let any negative thoughts or feelings swirl away.

Set the table. In our go-go-go world, we often eat while doing a million other things, like scrolling our phones or driving from place to place. We're probably not paying attention to the food so we're almost certainly not tasting or savoring it. Setting a table encourages you to slow down. You'll be primed to notice the textures, smells, and flavors of what you're eating. This attention will help increase your sense of taste, which is related to your sacral chakra. You'll simultaneously nourish your body, heighten your pleasure, and benefit your sacral chakra.

Journal Prompts

- What brings you pleasure? Be as specific as possible.
- What is your favorite form of artistic expression?
- Do you think of yourself as a creative person? Why or why not?
- When and where are you most in the flow?
- Describe a time when you used creativity to solve a problem.
- Why does balancing your sacral chakra matter to you at this moment?

SACRAL CHAKRA AT A GLANCE	
SANSKRIT NAME	Svadhishthana (sva-dish-tah-nah)
SYMBOL	Lotus flower with six petals
LOCATION	2 inches (5 cm) below the belly button
THIS CHAKRA IS CONNECTED TO	Being in the flow, creativity, pleasure, sensuality
COLOR	Orange
CRYSTALS	Amber, carnelian, citrine, moonstone, orange calcite
ELEMENT	Water
MANTRA	Vam
"I FEEL" AFFIRMATION	I feel joyful
ANIMAL	Crocodile
BENEFITS OF BALANCING THIS CHAKRA	Capacity for joy, emotional self-control, enhanced creativity, enthusiasm, playfulness
WHEN UNBALANCED	Jealousy, lack of passion or interest, lethargy, melancholy, mood swings

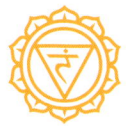

Solar Plexus Chakra

The solar plexus chakra is located between your navel and your breastbone, in the middle of your torso and beneath your rib cage. No doubt you've felt that area activate before—maybe as you did sit-ups, causing your ab muscles to strengthen and your posture to improve. Maybe you've felt butterflies fluttering right there, a sign of nervousness, or as if a heavy rock were lodged in your belly, a sure sign of dread. When we're impassioned, we talk about being "on fire" or "fired up," and those feelings also seem to emanate from this general region. If you put your hand there now, what would you feel?

The solar plexus chakra relates to how you present yourself to the world—confidently or otherwise. It's also affiliated with your ability to handle and deal with whatever the world hands you. It influences our sense of self, our personality, and our will or drive. This chakra gives us energy.

In Sanskrit, *manipura* means "lustrous gem" or "city of jewels." Thinking that we hold a jewel within us almost immediately improves our belief in ourselves. We go from feeling apprehensive to feeling proud, from being unsure to being brave. Thanks to the solar plexus chakra, our self-worth shoots up. We believe that we deserve the good things that have come, or are coming, to us. We have pluck and spunk.

WHY BALANCING YOUR SOLAR PLEXUS CHAKRA MATTERS

Without bravery, you can't live your authentic life. Without courage, you can't explore your passions or fulfill your purpose. Without a healthy ego, you can't be you, with all your signature talents and lovable quirks. Without energy, you'll have trouble doing much of anything, including setting and achieving goals. Without a balanced solar plexus chakra, you'll struggle with identity, drive, and fortitude.

The solar plexus chakra gets at the very core of who we are. It sits almost at the center of the body, and affects digestion. This chakra helps us cope with and handle what comes along. Without getting overly graphic, we take what we need—food or otherwise—and expel what we don't.

But the solar plexus chakra also influences how we deal with others. An inflated ego, for example, might try to manipulate people into doing what it wants, blindly pursuing its desires without consideration or care. Balanced, however, a solar plexus chakra offers the right amount of self-belief—that is, we have enough ego to help us cultivate ambition and be our true selves without steamrolling anyone else. Confident in ourselves, we assist and support others in achieving their goals.

What an Unbalanced Solar Plexus Chakra Feels Like

Too much internal fire turns us aggressive and angry. We lower our heads and charge, regardless of consequences. Our egos expand. Raging and out of control, this inflated sense of self-worth begins to consume everything in its path. A person with an overstimulated solar plexus chakra stops considering others and does whatever they want to do. All arrogance and dominance, tons of competitiveness, zero empathy, not a lick of thoughtfulness, etc.

Not enough internal fire turns us insecure, leading to feelings of inferiority and indecision. We stop believing in ourselves, so we stop setting goals, pursuing passions, and trying to live the life we want. Without the will to be productive, we lose stamina and discipline. Instead of standing straight, with a proud chest, we hunch or hide—literally, metaphorically, or both.

The solar plexus chakra is related to the gut. Physically, when our solar plexus chakra is unbalanced, we may experience digestive issues—from bloating to heartburn to cramps. Our stomach gets upset. Eating, of course, gives us energy in the form of calories. If we don't eat enough, for whatever reason, we become increasingly listless and our internal flame grows feeble.

UNBALANCED SOLAR PLEXUS CHAKRA	
PHYSICAL AILMENTS	MENTAL AND EMOTIONAL AILMENTS
Stomach cramps	Egotism
Bloating	Self-doubt
Nausea	Aggression
Disordered eating	Lack of willpower
Weak core	Passivity

How to Balance Your Solar Plexus Chakra

A balanced solar plexus chakra spurs our desire to set goals, supports the drive to pursue them, and stokes the confidence that comes from believing in ourselves. With the help of the solar plexus chakra, we are motivated to carve out the life we want.

Visualizations and Meditations

Spin the wheel. Envision a yellow wheel immediately beneath your rib cage, at the upper abdomen. Use your breath to make this wheel spin, or pace your breaths to its movement. As you watch the wheel turn, notice any sensations. Let yourself feel confident, capable, courageous, and certain.

Meditate on the color yellow. Picture a freshly cut pineapple, just-peeled banana, or newly opened yellow rose. Visualizing joyful yellow things—like a bursting sunflower, frolicking golden retriever, or tall glass of lemonade—can help you unlock your solar plexus chakra. Wearing an item of yellow clothing can help, too, as can wearing your chakra bracelet.

Fan your internal flames. If you've ever heard the expression "fire in the belly," you're on your way to accomplishing this visualization. The solar plexus chakra can spur us to productivity. Imagine a lovely, cozy fire beneath your rib cage. Feel the soothing heat of the flames, which might be yellow, red, orange, or even blue and white. Allow the fire's heat to move through you, warming and invigorating your limbs.

Uncover your passion. This meditation asks you to close your eyes and look deep into yourself and honestly answer the question, *What do I want from life?* Figuring this out takes time so don't get down on yourself if nothing pops up. Keep closing your eyes, relaxing, and asking. Relatedly, don't judge yourself if you answer the question differently from what you were expecting, or from how you answered it in the past. Discovering your passion gives direction and purpose to your drive so you can make your amazing energy work for you.

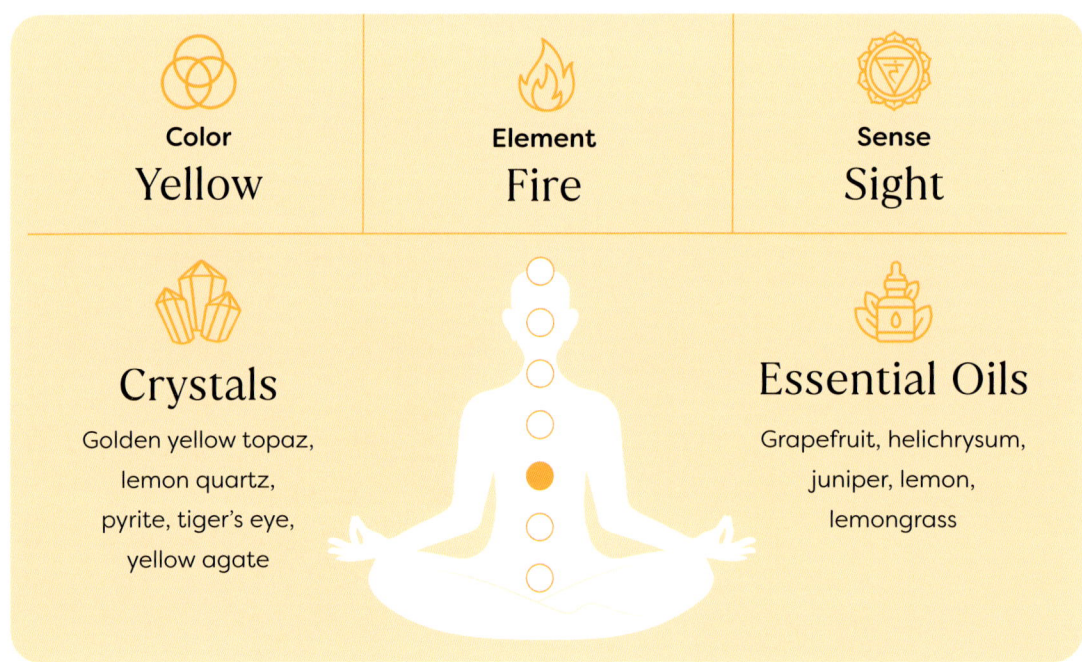

Color
Yellow

Element
Fire

Sense
Sight

Crystals
Golden yellow topaz, lemon quartz, pyrite, tiger's eye, yellow agate

Essential Oils
Grapefruit, helichrysum, juniper, lemon, lemongrass

Food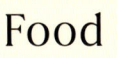

Fiber-rich foods like leafy greens and whole grains aid digestion and help keep the solar plexus chakra functioning at an optimal level. Fermented foods like kimchi, kombucha, and kefir also improve your gut's overall health (and keep things moving). Sipping peppermint or ginger tea can soothe an upset stomach.

Herbs and Spices

Clove, fennel, ginger, peppermint, turmeric

Yoga Poses and Stretches

Bow pose, seated spinal twist, supine spinal twist, upward-facing dog, wind-relieving pose

Breathwork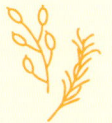

BREATH OF FIRE

Also referred to as *kapalabhati* or "skull shining breath," breath of fire powers you up and strengthens your core. It involves making quick, rapid exhales while pumping your belly toward your spine. Go slowly at first, then work up to practicing this breath for a full minute. Keep your hands on your knees, or put your hands on your stomach to feel it move.

1. Sit comfortably.
2. Move your shoulders away from your ears. Relax.
3. Inhale deeply through the nose.
4. Exhale short, sharp breaths through the nose. Exhalations should be rapid, even noisy.

5. Snap your belly to your spine on each exhale. It might take a few rounds to quicken your exhales, or to find a rhythm that works for your belly and breath. Your inhales will happen naturally.
6. Repeat for 30 seconds–1 minute, quickening your exhales as you go.
7. Resume breathing normally.

BREATH OF JOY

Like breath of fire, breath of joy infuses you with energy and enthusiasm. Avoid this breathwork technique if you have blood-pressure issues or are prone to migraines. Otherwise, try this practice when you start to feel sluggish or apathetic.

1. Stand up straight with your feet about shoulder-width apart. Bend your knees slightly.
2. Move your shoulders away from your ears. Relax.
3. Inhale through your nose while raising your arms to shoulder height.
4. While hinging forward at the waist as far forward as feels comfortable, exhale, letting your arms swing behind you.
5. Inhale to straighten, raising your arms in front of you. Keep them at shoulder height, or raise them above your head.
6. Exhale and hinge.
7. Repeat a few times, but beware of becoming lightheaded.
8. Resume breathing normally.

Mantra Chant Sound

Ram (pronounced *ruuummm*)

Flowers and Plants

Daffodil, evening primrose, forsythia, Shasta daisy, sunflower

Affirmations

I am brave.
I have done hard things, and I can do hard things.
I am willing to try new things.
I believe in myself.
I have the energy to accomplish everything that matters to me.

Acts of Service

Share your knowledge. Putting yourself forward as a knowledgeable source requires bravery as well as confidence, two traits affiliated with the solar plexus chakra. You must believe in yourself enough to feel you can impart worthwhile information to another. But you don't need to stand in front of a classroom to teach—you can do so in a less formal way, such as offering tips to a friend who's starting an activity you've mastered. All the better if you can position yourself as a teacher who's also a student, willing to walk alongside others at different stages of the learning journey.

Be a cheerleader. Setting goals is often the easy part; achieving them is what's hard. Pick someone in your life who is working toward accomplishing a goal, and who could use some motivation and support. How can you cheer them on? With their permission, you might schedule regular check-ins, join them for an activity (such as a quick walk, if their goal is to get healthy, for example), or help them brainstorm ways to make a big project more manageable. Encouraging someone else will assist your solar plexus chakra by emphasizing the power of motivation and self-belief.

Everyday Activities to Activate Your Solar Plexus Chakra

Light a candle. A balanced solar plexus chakra is like a little sun we carry within us, providing power and vitality. We're inspired, and we're on fire in the best possible way. You can access this feeling by lighting a candle, which brings warmth into your space. For an added benefit to your solar plexus chakra, pick an invigorating scent, like lemongrass eucalyptus. Lighting a fire in a fireplace or firepit works, too. As you contemplate the flame, think about co-opting its energy and powering yourself up.

Do some cardio. Runners often talk about a "runner's high," or the feeling of exhilaration that results from exercise. But you don't need to run to get the same boost of positive hormones and activation of your solar plexus chakra. Walking, jogging, swimming, aerobicizing, jumping rope, and skipping down the block all work—the key is to move your body to the point where it's difficult to carry on a conversation. Do that regularly, and you'll see higher levels of energy, an improved mood, and enhanced confidence.

Self-Care Rituals for Your Solar Plexus Chakra

Meal prep. Imagine coming home after a long day, only to open your freezer and discover . . . delicious frozen meals you made the week before. Prepping food for yourself makes it easy to maintain healthy eating habits—and can be a powerful act of self-care. It's one of the ways You Right Now can appreciate and take care of Future You.

Pare down your to-do list. Time is a finite resource. If we say yes to everything, we might find ourselves stretched too thin or unable to finish what we agreed to do. Instead of adding to your list, consider what to delegate or decline. A streamlined list will not only improve your ability to focus (which also helps your third eye chakra), it might also make you excited to dive in.

Engage your core. More than your abs, your core is the entire group of muscles linking your upper and lower halves, including back, hips, pelvis, and side body. A strong core helps you stand and sit up straight, thereby projecting a proud self to the world (and tuning your solar plexus chakra). As you move about your day, tighten your navel to your spine (no slouching or hunching!).

Journal Prompts

- What's your proudest achievement to date?
- What's one thing you do better than anyone else?
- What gives you confidence?
- Describe a time when you showed tremendous bravery or courage.
- What's an activity you've always wanted to try?
- What's stopping you from trying it?
- Why does balancing your solar plexus chakra matter to you at this moment?

SOLAR PLEXUS CHAKRA AT A GLANCE	
SANSKRIT NAME	Manipura (mahn-ee-pur-ah)
SYMBOL	Lotus flower with ten petals
LOCATION	Middle of the torso, between the navel and breastbone
THIS CHAKRA IS CONNECTED TO	Confidence, drive, self-worth, strength
COLOR	Yellow
CRYSTALS	Golden yellow topaz, lemon quartz, pyrite, tiger's eye, yellow agate
ELEMENT	Fire
MANTRA	Ram
"I FEEL" AFFIRMATION	I feel confident and strong
ANIMAL	Ram
BENEFITS OF BALANCING THIS CHAKRA	Ambition, bravery, confidence, courage, energy, increased self-confidence
WHEN UNBALANCED	Aggression, digestion issues, lassitude, low self-esteem, timidity

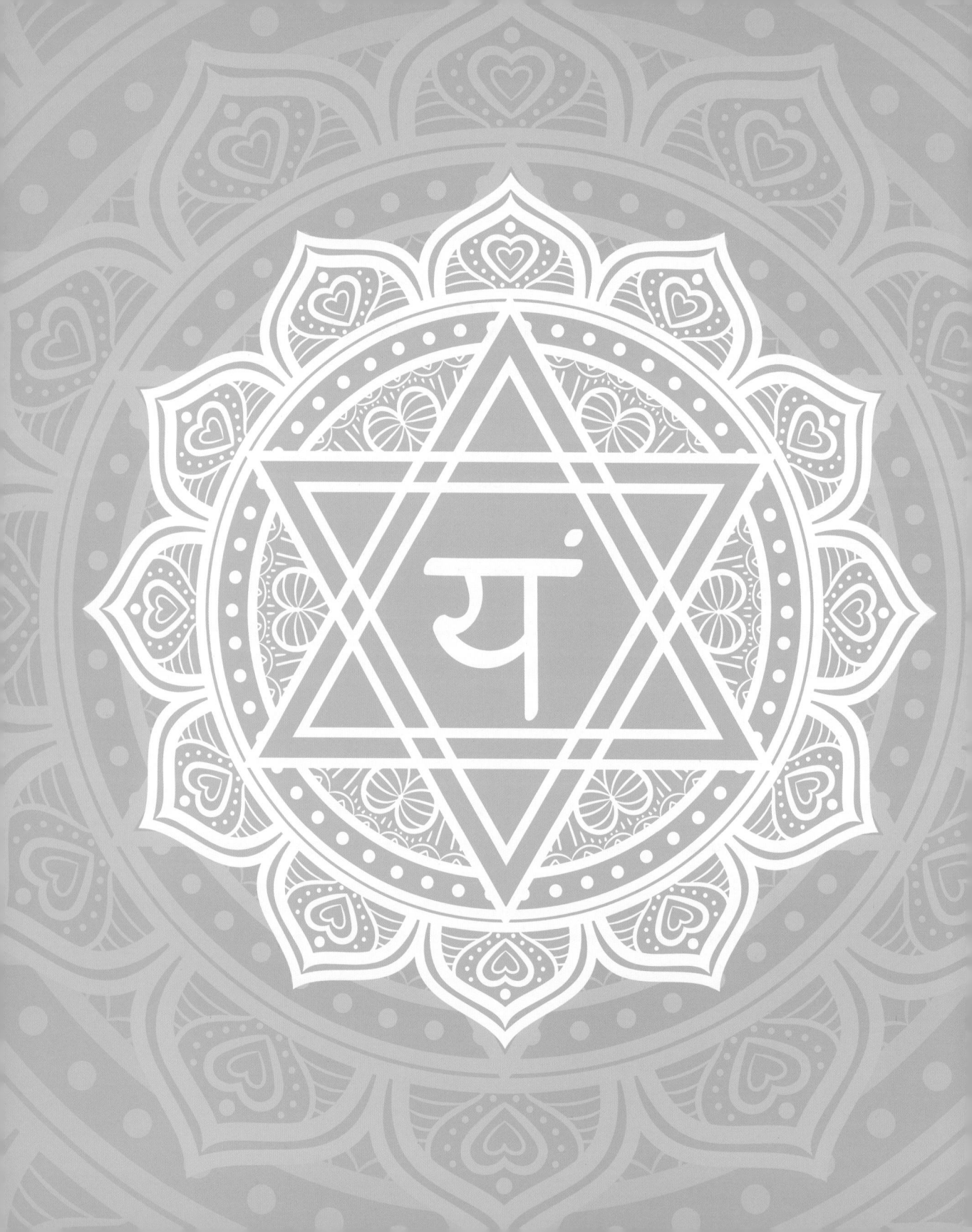

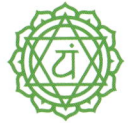

Heart Chakra

In the chakra system, the heart chakra is located in the center of the chest. Like your physical heart, which is slightly to the left, the heart chakra is affiliated with love, empathy, gratitude, and compassion. Unbalanced, we're curmudgeonly and bitter—Ebenezer Scrooge before the redemption, or Ron Swanson without Leslie Knope.

The heart chakra acts as a bridge between those chakras that are more oriented toward the physical (root, sacral, solar plexus) and those that are more oriented toward the cerebral and the spiritual (throat, third eye, crown). Some wellness experts see affiliations between the heart chakra and the vagus nerve, the body's large nerve system that acts like an information superhighway between the brain, heart, and digestive system.

However, we can work on opening our hearts. The Sanskrit word for the heart chakra, *anahata*, is usually translated as "unstruck" and "unhurt." When we love and are loved in return, we're at peace, unstruck and unstuck. Scientists have discovered that people in romantic relationships will often mimic one another's heartbeats—a verifiable demonstration of the giving and receiving of loving energy.

Along with the heart, the heart chakra is connected to the body's immune system, which helps us stay well and disease-free (unhurt). The heart chakra, likewise, relates to our ability to heal, including from heartbreak and grief.

WHY BALANCING YOUR HEART CHAKRA MATTERS

A person with a balanced heart chakra radiates warmth. They give great hugs, and they make their loved ones feel seen and heard. If someone in their orbit messes up, a balanced heart chakra will help this person assume good intent and forgive easily. Their well of compassion never seems to run dry. Instead, in their eyes, all of us are better versions of ourselves.

Love is among the most powerful of feelings. When we truly love ourselves, we make good choices and act thoughtfully, avoiding situations that might be bad or unhealthy for us. When we love other people—and keep that love top of mind—we consider their feelings and do what we can to support, honor, and appreciate them.

Too often, though, we forget, and the immediacy or sense of love falls away. We start to take each other or ourselves for granted. We make the poor choice, speak sharply, or act without thinking. A balanced heart chakra brings our awareness back to the fundamentals: love, joy, compassion, kindness—to ourselves, to others, to our planet, and to all those who inhabit it.

What an Unbalanced Heart Chakra Feels Like

If you don't love yourself, you can't love anyone else. You might be critical and judgmental toward yourself and those around you. An underactive heart chakra closes off our hearts. Without love in our lives, we become increasingly lonely, isolated, and alienated. We resent others, turning bitter and angry, which pushes connection even farther away. Neglecting this chakra can transform the most extroverted among us into growlers and grumps.

An overactive chakra can lead to people-pleasing. In this state, we might do anything to be loved, including lowering or dismissing our boundaries. Although we want to charm and bring joy to those around us, an unhealthy desire to make someone else happy can erase one's sense of self (which also damages the solar plexus chakra). This extreme focus on others could also lead to jealousy and possessiveness, as when we start to resent when a loved one hangs out with or shows affection to someone else.

The heart chakra reminds us of the fine line between wanting to feel loved by others and needing someone else's love in order to feel complete.

UNBALANCED HEART CHAKRA	
PHYSICAL AILMENTS	MENTAL AND EMOTIONAL AILMENTS
Shoulder pain	Fault-finding
Upper-back pain	Lack of empathy
Poor circulation	Isolation
Heart palpitations	Negative self-talk
Shortness of breath	Possessiveness

How to Balance Your Heart Chakra

Exercise and touch are two ways we can boost our body's production of oxytocin, sometimes called the "love hormone." Not surprisingly, high levels of this hormone lead to feelings of well-being as well as feelings of affection and attraction. Plus oxytocin has been shown to help heal our heart, all of which benefits our heart chakra.

Visualizations and Meditations

Spin the wheel. Envision a green wheel at the center of your chest. Use your breath to make this wheel spin, or pace your breaths to its movement. As you watch the wheel turn, notice any sensations. Let yourself feel loved and give love in return.

Meditate on the color green. Picture a lush lawn, ripe green apple, or your favorite park at the height of summer. Visualizing joyful green things—like a just-cut honeydew melon, cushy layer of pine needles on the forest floor, or bunch of fresh parsley—can help you unlock your heart chakra. Wearing an item of green clothing can help, too, as can wearing your chakra bracelet.

Practice the loving-kindness meditation. There are many variations on this well-known meditation, each of which sends love into the world. This meditation can be done anytime, anywhere. If you're alone, conjure the face of someone you'd like to send love to, such as a friend in need or someone with whom you've had challenges. If you're out and about, silently recite the meditation and beam its benefits to a stranger, secretly and unselfishly. The following version consists of four simple phrases, repeated sequentially:

May you be happy.
May you be healthy.
May you be peaceful.
May you be protected.

Envelop yourself in a bubble of love. When we love ourselves, we set healthy boundaries. This visualization helps create a positive, protective barrier between you and the rest of the world. Begin by sitting quietly, with your eyes closed. As you start to relax into your breath, imagine a beautiful bubble developing around you. Feel free to pick a color that pleases you, although you might consider green, the color of the heart chakra. Let it grow stronger with each breath you take. When you feel ready, open your eyes, but keep the bubble enveloping you as you move through the world.

THE SEVEN MAJOR CHAKRAS | HEART CHAKRA

Color
Green

Element
Air

Sense
Touch

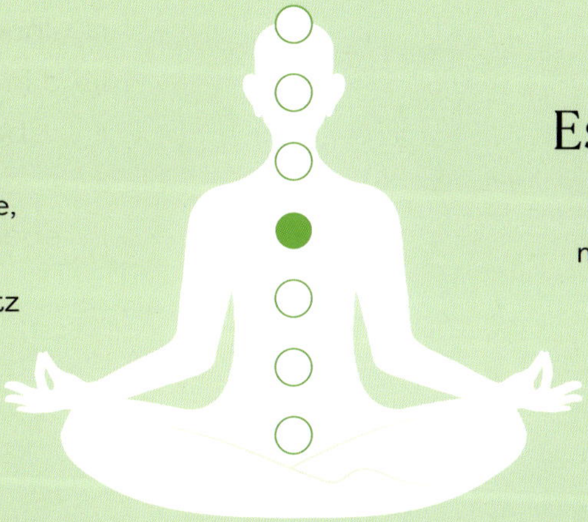

Crystals
Emerald, moss agate, pink tourmaline, rhodonite, rose quartz

Essential Oils
Cypress, geranium, marjoram, pine, rose

Food

Significant food choices we can make for our heart chakra are those that help our heart, such as olive oil and legumes. We can opt for green foods like avocado. But perhaps the best means of helping this chakra is by eating a meal cooked with love. It's a magical, free ingredient that nourishes us on a deep spiritual level.

THE SEVEN MAJOR CHAKRAS | HEART CHAKRA

Herbs and Spices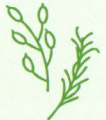

Basil, cayenne pepper, celery seed, cilantro, garlic

Yoga Poses and Stretches

Bridge/wheel, cat-cow, cobra pose, dancer's pose, fish pose

Breathwork

BOX BREATH

Also known as "square" or "paced breathing," this technique evens out your inhales and exhales. Developed by a former US Navy SEAL, box breath has been shown to reduce stress, combat insomnia, and increase focus; it's also thought to increase lung capacity. You can do it sitting, standing, or lying down—pretty much anywhere, anytime. If holding your breath after inhaling or exhaling makes you uncomfortable, skip it and instead focus on pacing your inhales and exhales to a slow count of four.

1. Lie flat, sit comfortably, or stand up straight.
2. Move your shoulders away from your ears. Relax.
3. Inhale through your nose for four counts.
4. Hold your breath for four counts.
5. Exhale for four counts.
6. Pause for four counts.
7. Inhale, starting the sequence again. If a count of four seems like too much, aim for a count of two or three.
8. Repeat for a few cycles, or until you feel calm and focused.
9. Resume breathing normally.

PURSED-LIP BREATH

Exhaling through pursed lips has been shown to increase lung capacity, allowing more fresh air to enter your lungs, which helps people breathe better overall. As with belly breathing (see pages 29–30) or box breath, you can do this breathwork sitting, standing, or lying down, whenever you need to pause and center yourself. Try to exhale slowly and with control, to make your exhalations longer than your inhalations (aim for your exhales to be double the length of your inhales), and to empty your lungs on each exhalation.

1. Lie flat, sit comfortably, or stand up straight.
2. Move your shoulders away from your ears. Relax.
3. Inhale through your nose for as long as feels comfortable.
4. Exhale through your mouth, pursing your lips as if you were sipping from a straw. Unlike belly breathing, your goal here is to let all the air out of your lungs.
5. Repeat for three to five complete cycles.
6. Resume breathing normally.

Mantra Chant Sound

Yam (pronounced *yuuummm*)

Affirmations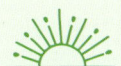

I am loved.
I give and receive love.
The power of love dwells within me.
I feel love and compassion for all living things.
I deserve love.

Flowers and Plants

Carnation, clematis, heartleaf philodendron, rubber plant, sweetheart plant

Acts of Service

Tackle someone's (dreaded) chore. The business of life involves all manner of unpleasant tasks, from cleaning out gutters to filing one's taxes. As an act of service for someone you love, consider performing a task they've been dreading or putting off for whatever reason. Lightening their load will certainly surround you both with positive feelings, and just might invigorate you enough to turn to a chore of your own.

Participate enthusiastically. Although we love our friends or romantic partner, we may not always love their hobbies. As an act of service that shows your love—and affects your heart chakra—offer to participate in an activity they adore that you might not adore so much. Each of us feels loved, and expresses love, in different ways—and, as much as we love someone, sometimes we don't show it in quite the right way. Here's your chance to say yes to the joint cooking class, to the live Formula 1 event, to attending a marathon reading of *Moby Dick*. If your person is into it, you can be into it for an afternoon, too. Then, if you're lucky, your friend or partner will spend time returning the favor and doing something you love.

Everyday Activities to Activate Your Heart Chakra

Read a novel. Fiction has been shown to increase empathy, leading researchers to conclude that reading novels can make us better people. The more transported we are by a book, the more we care about the characters, the more we carry such feelings of compassion into our daily lives. Empathy forms a cornerstone of an open heart chakra, as it enables us to sympathize with and be loving toward those around us.

Have a cuddle. Positive, consensual touch has been shown to reduce depression, lower one's heart rate, increase feelings of safety, and decrease anxiety. Conversely, touch deprivation causes many negative effects, including heightened aggression. Because the heart chakra is related to touch and skin, massage, hugging, and yoga (a form of self-touch) can soothe it, as can interacting with an animal.

Answer the phone. Or text or email. If someone reaches out, take the time to reach back. Don't underestimate the power of a quick check-in to help strengthen your relationships, bring more love into your life, and balance your heart chakra. Chatting for a few minutes also spares you from having to engage in a series of back-and-forths about scheduling or from wondering when you might have time to return the call.

Self-Care Rituals for Your Heart Chakra

Do something nice for yourself. Buy yourself flowers, or skip cooking and order takeout. Make your bed. Spend an hour reading a book or watching a favorite show. Go through the pictures on your phone, then get some printed to hang on your refrigerator or to put into frames. Eat some ice cream, do some pull-ups, make a playlist of songs you used to love but haven't heard in a while. Call an old friend. Almost any activity will do for your heart chakra as long as it helps self-love bloom.

Lower the volume on your inner critic. Each of us has an inner critic. Too often, we let this inner critic speak to us in ways we'd never tolerate from anyone else. In fact, sometimes we turn up the volume and tune in, as if this bully were a beloved podcast. Of course, holding yourself to a high standard matters, and an inner critic can guide you toward smart choices. However, if it's all you hear, you need to cultivate self-compassion ASAP. Talk to yourself as you would to a friend, with kindness and sensitivity. If you wouldn't say it to someone else, why say it to yourself?

THE SEVEN MAJOR CHAKRAS | HEART CHAKRA

Journal Prompts

- *What do you love most about yourself?*
- *What is your favorite way to show love?*
- *Write about a time when you showed yourself genuine compassion and self-love.*
- *Describe a moment when you felt truly seen and loved by someone else.*
- *What does unconditional love mean to you?*
- *Why does balancing your heart chakra matter to you at this moment?*

HEART CHAKRA AT A GLANCE	
SANSKRIT NAME	Anahata (ah-nah-hah-tah)
SYMBOL	Lotus flower with twelve petals
LOCATION	Center of the chest
THIS CHAKRA IS CONNECTED TO	Compassion, empathy, love and friendship, self-love
COLOR	Green
CRYSTALS	Emerald, moss agate, pink tourmaline, rhodonite, rose quartz
ELEMENT	Air
MANTRA	Yam
"I FEEL" AFFIRMATION	I feel loved
ANIMAL	Antelope
BENEFITS OF BALANCING THIS CHAKRA	Compassion, empathy, forgiveness, love for others, self-love
WHEN UNBALANCED	Bitterness, criticism, disgruntlement, emotional isolation, lack of boundaries

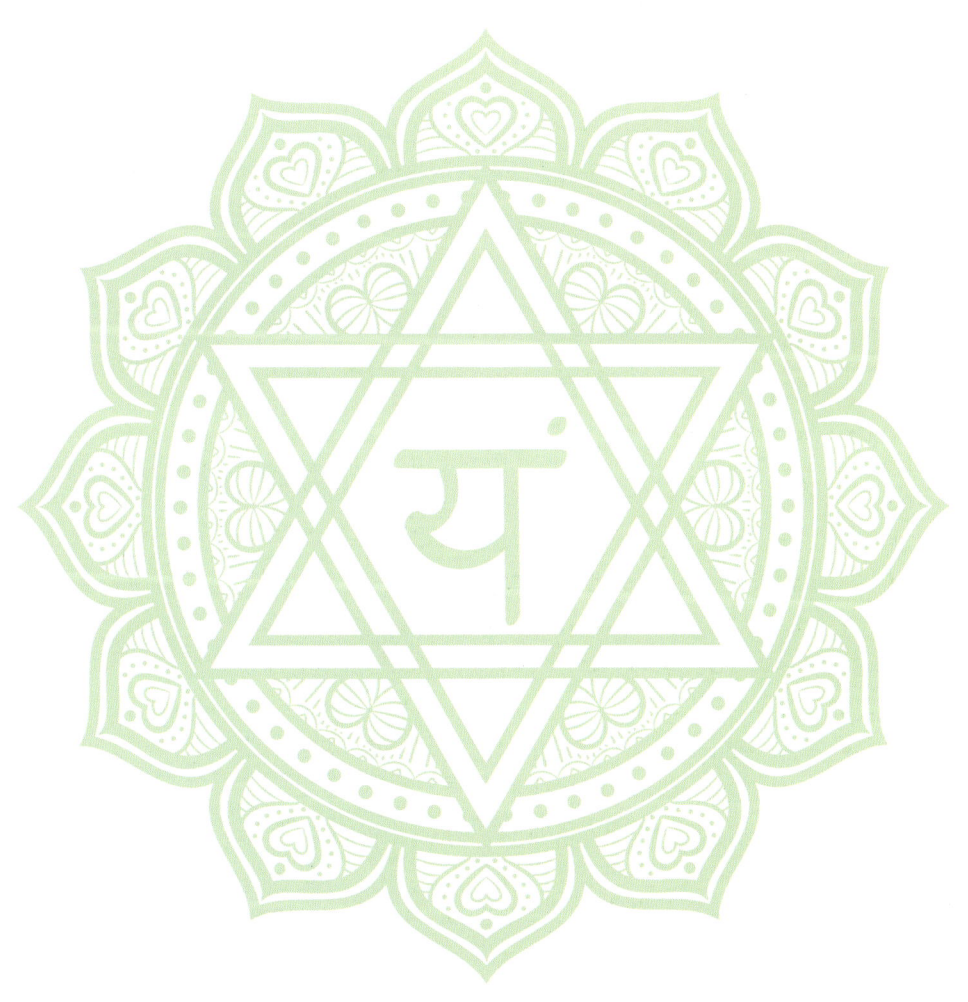

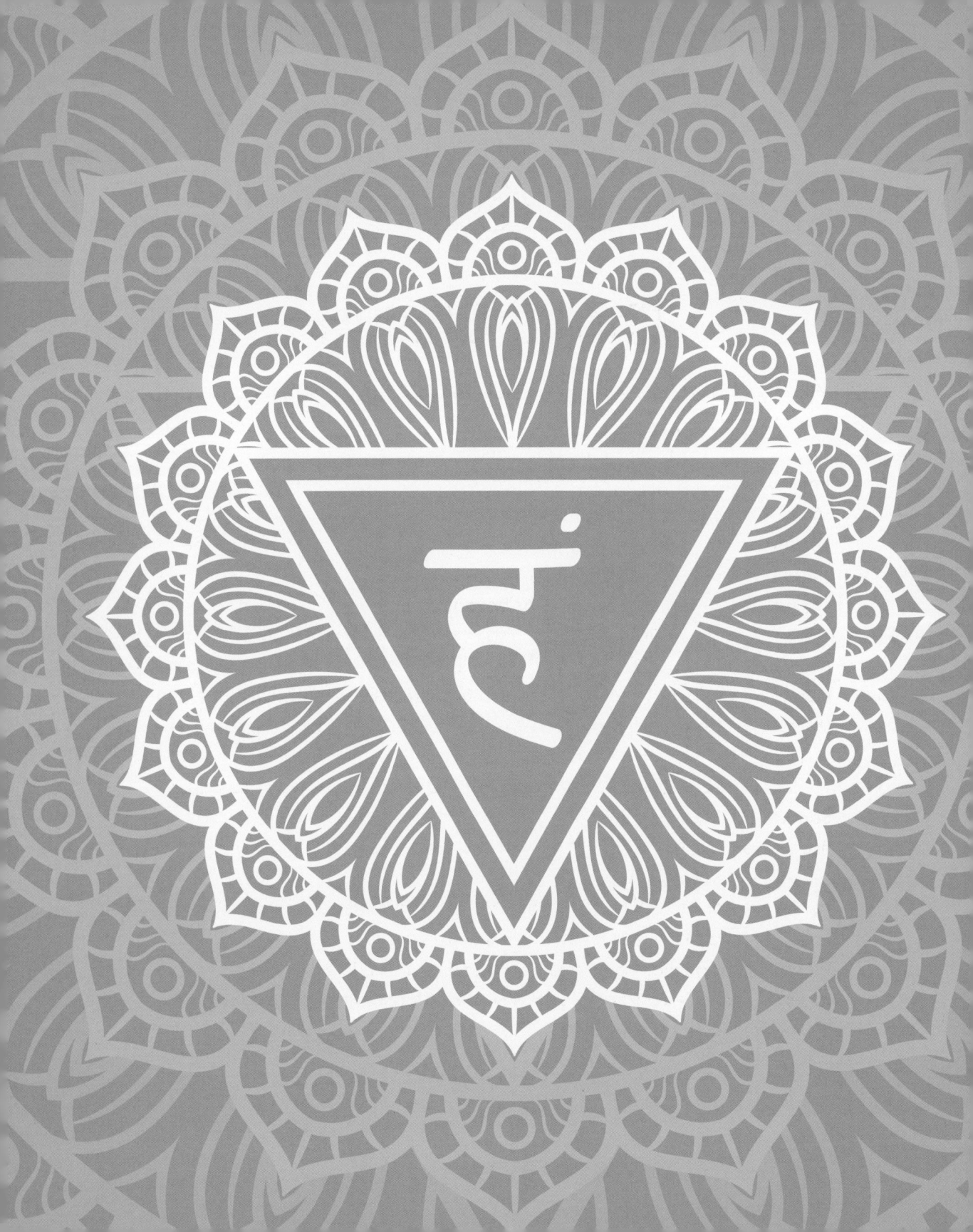

Throat Chakra

You've probably heard the phrase "speaking one's truth." When we use this phrase, we're really talking about being able to communicate honestly and openly. We can share our hopes, fears, boundaries, wants, and needs. As important, we feel confident that such expressions will be heard and understood by others. Located at the base of the throat, the throat chakra is concerned with our ability to use our voice in this way—and when aligned, encourages us to speak our truth.

But the throat chakra extends beyond self-expression. Being a good communicator means learning to listen and encourage someone else to express themselves. It means asking the right questions and fostering a demeanor that welcomes dialogue, rather than lectures or monologues. By the same token, having a powerful voice means using your words to uplift and support others.

Speaking one's truth also means living authentically and with integrity. In Sanskrit, the throat chakra is called *vishuddha*, generally translated as "purification" or "especially pure." A person who has to hide some aspect of themselves won't feel as if they're living a pure life.

Along with the physical throat, the throat chakra oversees the teeth, jaw, mouth, and shoulders. When we wish to hide, we hunch our shoulders. When forced to hold our tongue, we might clench our jaw or mash our teeth together. When we're anxious or upset, our throat closes up. Aligning the throat chakra can mitigate these physical and emotional responses.

WHY BALANCING YOUR THROAT CHAKRA MATTERS

A balanced throat chakra teaches us to admit when we're wrong. We're able to use our words to help and heal, not to hurt someone or hide the truth. Our voice is a force for good. We don't speak without thought, nor do we talk to fill the air. What we say matters.

The throat chakra is also associated with having a large vocabulary. The more words we know, the more we're able to describe a situation or a feeling with precision—and the more likely it is that someone will understand what we're trying to say and that our message will be received. A balanced throat chakra enables us to avoid miscommunication and to speak our minds passionately, accurately, and appropriately.

Our actions reflect our words. Put another way: In addition to speaking our truth authentically, we act in ways that are true to ourselves. The throat chakra connects to our moral compass. We don't traffic in secrets. We live with integrity and authenticity. By valuing honesty, we encourage others to be honest with us by being honest in every facet of our life.

What an Unbalanced Throat Chakra Feels Like

An unbalanced throat chakra leads to communication blockages of all kinds, including an inability to express yourself verbally or creatively. You can't or don't want to talk, nor do you feel like listening to yourself or anyone else. Words get bitten back, and emotions are swallowed. You feel inauthentic, like you're living someone else's life rather than your own, or playing a part full of lines you haven't memorized.

Sometimes, instead of shutting down one's powers of communication, an unbalanced throat chakra turns them hyper. A person may lie, almost pathologically, making up truths they wish were real. They may gossip, spread rumors, or become know-it-alls. Too busy nattering and blathering, they cease to pay attention to what they or anyone else is saying. Words might be expressed, but the words lack meaning or substance. These people talk and talk but say nothing.

An underactive throat chakra can lead to whininess or shyness. Despite a wish to be heard, the lack of energetic activity within this chakra prevents you from using your voice. Inarticulate, you become fearful of expressing your glorious, wonderful, unique self (which affects your sacral and solar plexus chakras as well).

UNBALANCED THROAT CHAKRA	
PHYSICAL AILMENTS	MENTAL AND EMOTIONAL AILMENTS
Congestion	Poor listening
Sore throat	Self-censorship
Teeth grinding	Rumormongering
Neck pain	Know-it-all
Tooth decay and cavities	Long-windedness

How to Balance Your Throat Chakra

Simply rolling your neck a few times, or adjusting your posture to make sure your head is aligned with your shoulders, can ease your throat chakra. Other actions include singing, talking, and otherwise expressing yourself in healthy, even boisterous, ways. The throat chakra delights in open and genuine self-expression.

Visualizations and Meditations

Spin the wheel. Envision a blue wheel at the base of your throat. Use your breath to make this wheel spin, or pace your breaths to its movement. As you watch the wheel turn, notice any sensations. Let yourself feel tranquil, peaceful, and connected to your inner truth.

Meditate on the color blue. Picture a cloudless blue sky or placid lake. Visualizing joyful blue things—like a pod of blue whales, band of blue jays, or patch of blueberries—can help you unlock your throat chakra. Wearing an item of blue clothing can help, too, as can wearing your chakra bracelet.

Try a silent meditation. Our world is a noisy place. In this meditation, you simply sit in silence, letting your thoughts come and go. No judgment, no stress, no intention. When your mind wanders, patiently guide it back to your gentle inhales and exhales. Being silent for a while enables our throat chakra to rest—and, if we listen, we can start to hear a voice within us. What it has to say might surprise us.

Hum. A 2023 study found that the simple act of humming can activate the parasympathetic nervous system, thereby reducing stress. Sometimes called *bhramari* or "bee breathing," this meditation can be done anywhere. Inhale, then make a low hum as you exhale. Increase the intensity by shutting your eyes and plugging your ears with your thumbs, raising your elbows and resting your fingers lightly on your forehead. Feel the vibrations resonating from your throat, up through your head and down into your body.

THE SEVEN MAJOR CHAKRAS | THROAT CHAKRA

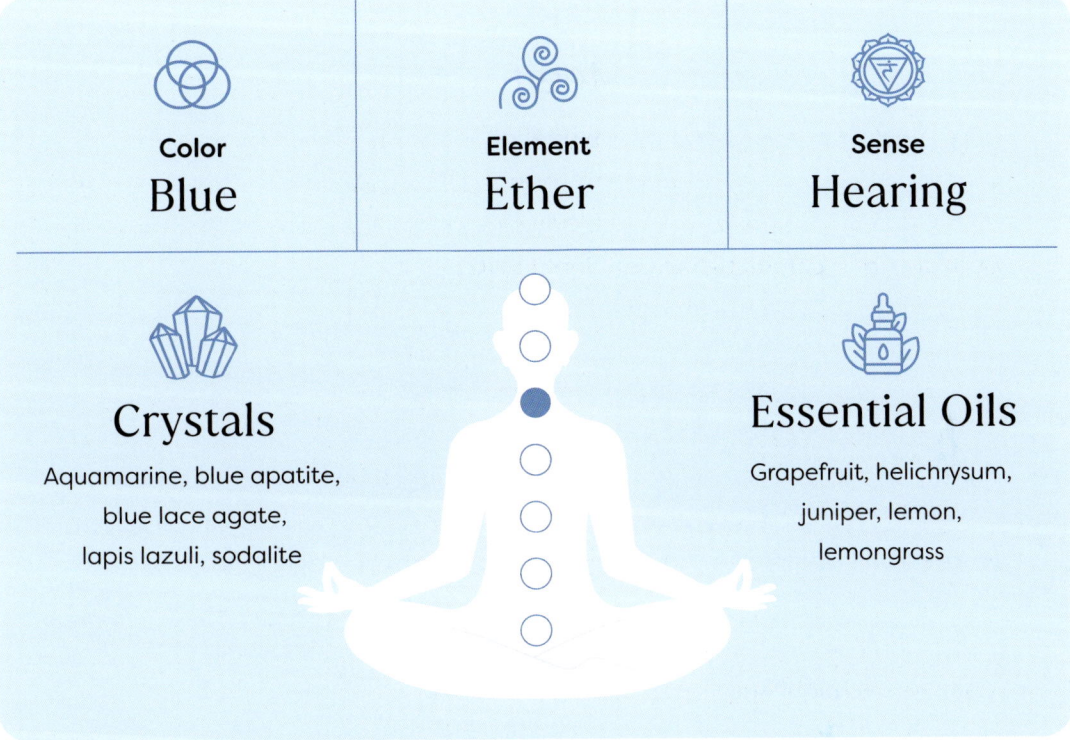

Color
Blue

Element
Ether

Sense
Hearing

Crystals
Aquamarine, blue apatite, blue lace agate, lapis lazuli, sodalite

Essential Oils
Grapefruit, helichrysum, juniper, lemon, lemongrass

Food

Start with foods that calm or comfort the throat, such as smoothies and soups. Add honey to your favorite tea, or take a spoonful straight to ease scratchiness and discomfort. Drink fruit juice or coconut water. Blue foods—such as blueberries, Concord grapes, and prunes (dried plums)—also help the throat chakra.

Herbs and Spices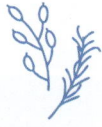

Dill, echinacea, elderberry, marshmallow root, slippery elm

Yoga Poses and Stretches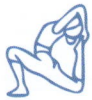

Camel pose, downward-facing dog, lion pose, plow pose, shoulder stand

Breathwork

LION'S BREATH

Lion's breath helps stimulate the throat by exercising your vocal cords and nearby muscles. This type of breathwork also encourages you to let go of any anxiety and bad feelings, kind of like the way we sometimes sigh or groan in exasperation before taking a deep breath and moving on.

1. Sit comfortably, kneel on all fours, or stand up straight.
2. Move your shoulders away from your ears. Relax.
3. Inhale through your nose.
4. Open your mouth and your eyes as wide as feels comfortable.
5. Stick out your tongue as you forcibly exhale. This exhale should sound like the roar of a lion.
6. Breathe normally for a few breaths, then do another round of lion's breath.
7. After at least five rounds of lion's breath, resume breathing normally.

UJJAYI BREATH

Also called "ocean breath," ujjayi breath involves constricting the throat and making a Darth Vader–like noise on the exhale. Some people liken this noisy exhale to the sound of ocean waves. Ujjayi breath is one of the most common types of *pranayama* (breathing regulation techniques) in yoga, and is used to improve concentration and increase relaxation.

1. Sit comfortably or stand up straight.
2. Move your shoulders away from your ears. Relax.
3. Inhale through your nose.

4. Exhale through your nose, but constrict your throat so you make a sound like a snore or the ocean. It might help to touch the tip of your tongue to the roof of your mouth.
5. Try to keep your inhales and exhales the same length.
6. Repeat for at least five cycles.
7. Resume breathing normally.

Mantra Chant Sound

Ham (pronounced *huummm*)

Affirmations

I am true to myself.
My insights and opinions matter.
I know when to speak and when to listen.
I trust myself and listen to my inner voice.
My words do no harm.

Flowers and Plants

Bluebell, blue iris, hyacinth, lithodora, starflower

Acts of Service

Listen actively. Too often, when we think we're listening, we're really just waiting quietly until it's our turn to speak. Listening not only allows you to honor the person with whom you're conversing, but it also gives you the chance to contribute meaningfully. What you say will be more impactful because you'll be responding to what someone else has said. And, perhaps, you might find you don't need to say anything at all. One of the most powerful acts of service we can undertake is to give our full attention to people when they speak, especially when that person happens to be sharing a perspective that's different from our own.

Befriend someone. When you're a kid, making new friends is easy—you're in the same class, plus you both like peanut butter–and–banana sandwiches. As you get older, though, making new friends gets harder, partly because there are fewer opportunities and partly because it can be awkward. But engaging with someone new requires you to be vulnerable and accept their vulnerabilities in return. True friendship blooms where there's authenticity and honesty. Being a false friend, with the attendant unbalanced throat chakra, won't get a person very far.

Everyday Activities to Activate Your Throat Chakra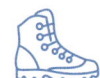

Sing. You don't have to be Taylor Swift to reap the benefits of singing. Studies have shown that singing enhances lung function for better breathing, increases the body's immune response, and strengthens its ability to withstand pain. When done in a group setting, singing has been shown to help synchronize people's heartbeats, thereby increasing social ties and decreasing loneliness (and benefiting the heart chakra, too). Last but not least, singing offers a powerful outlet for self-expression, allowing us to release emotions in a safe way (as anyone who's cranked up the music after a hard day can attest).

Take care of your teeth. Keep your chompers healthy by brushing twice a day and flossing at least once a day. See your dentist regularly for checkups and cleanings. No doubt you've been hearing such advice your entire life. What you might not know, however, is that oral health has been shown to significantly impact a person's overall health, given that the mouth and throat act as a gateway for bad bacteria into the rest of the body. In fact, poor dental hygiene correlates to a slew of other issues, including Alzheimer's disease, cardiovascular disease, and respiratory ailments. All the more reason to brush.

Self-Care Rituals for Your Throat Chakra

Journal. While writing out your thoughts and feelings can help with all the chakras, journaling is especially beneficial for the throat chakra. Expressing ourselves matters, but so does the means and manner by which we do so. That is, not every feeling or thought must be vocalized or articulated to another person; simply telling yourself is often enough. Journaling helps us discriminate between the truths we need to share with people in our lives and the truths we need to acknowledge to ourselves.

Make an herbal steam inhalation. Steam inhalations were first used by ancient Egyptians some 3,500 years ago. You can participate in this age-old remedy by heating 2 quarts (1.9 L) of water until steaming (not boiling), then adding two handfuls of fresh herbs, such as mint, sage, or thyme. Pour the mixture into a heatproof bowl. Cover your head with a towel to make a tent over the bowl and breathe in the steam for 10 minutes (max). Toss the herbal water afterward, or leave it out to help purify the air. Always be careful when handling or inhaling very hot water to avoid burns.

Journal Prompts

- *What are you feeling right now?*
- *When was the last time you felt heard and understood?*
- *Describe a time when you felt misunderstood.*
- *Write out a conversation you wish you could have with someone.*
- *What is the most meaningful thing anyone has ever said to you? What is the most meaningful thing you've ever said to someone else?*
- *Why does balancing your throat chakra matter to you at this moment?*

THE SEVEN MAJOR CHAKRAS | THROAT CHAKRA

THROAT CHAKRA AT A GLANCE	
SANSKRIT NAME	Vishuddha (vish-hood-he)
SYMBOL	Lotus flower with sixteen petals
LOCATION	Base of the throat
THIS CHAKRA IS CONNECTED TO	Authenticity, communication, truth
COLOR	Blue
CRYSTALS	Aquamarine, blue apatite, blue lace agate, lapis lazuli, sodalite
ELEMENT	Ether
MANTRA	Ham
"I FEEL" AFFIRMATION	I feel true to myself
ANIMAL	Lion
BENEFITS OF BALANCING THIS CHAKRA	Excellent communication skills, genuineness, integrity, self-awareness, self-expression
WHEN UNBALANCED	Bragging, dishonesty, exaggeration, misunderstandings, problems communicating

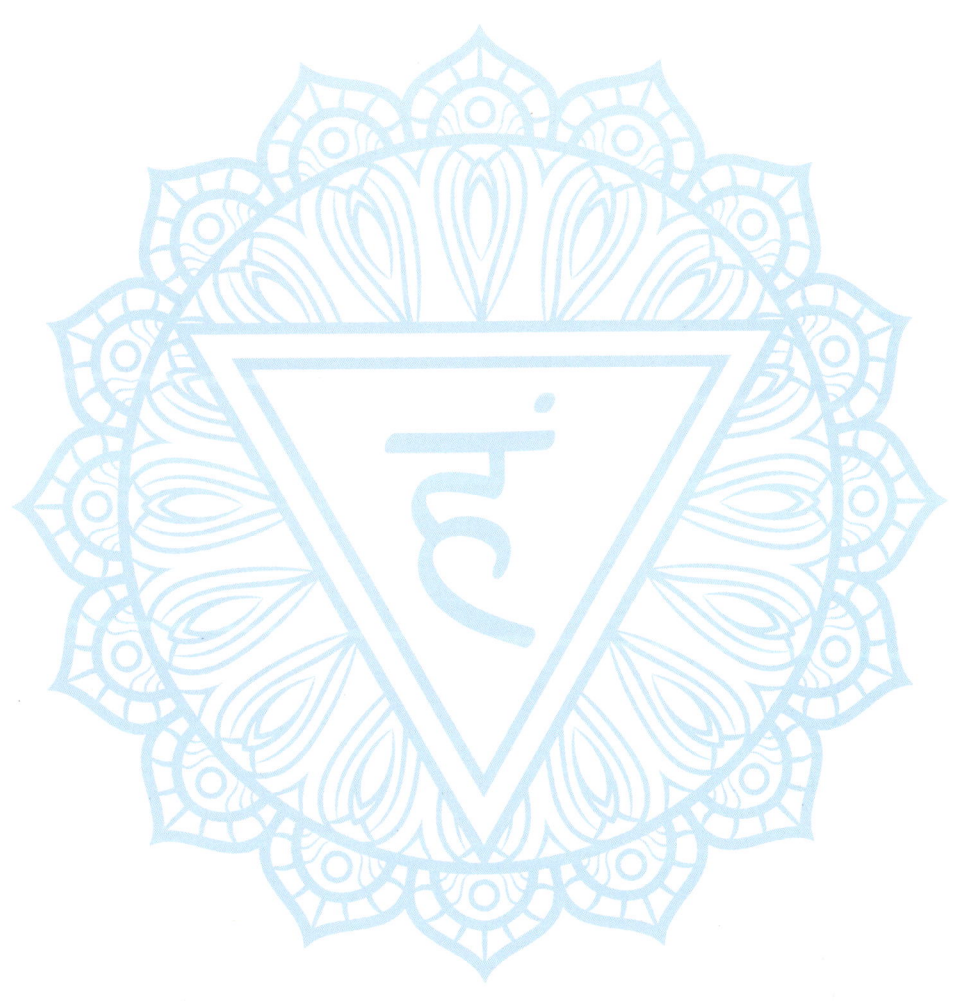

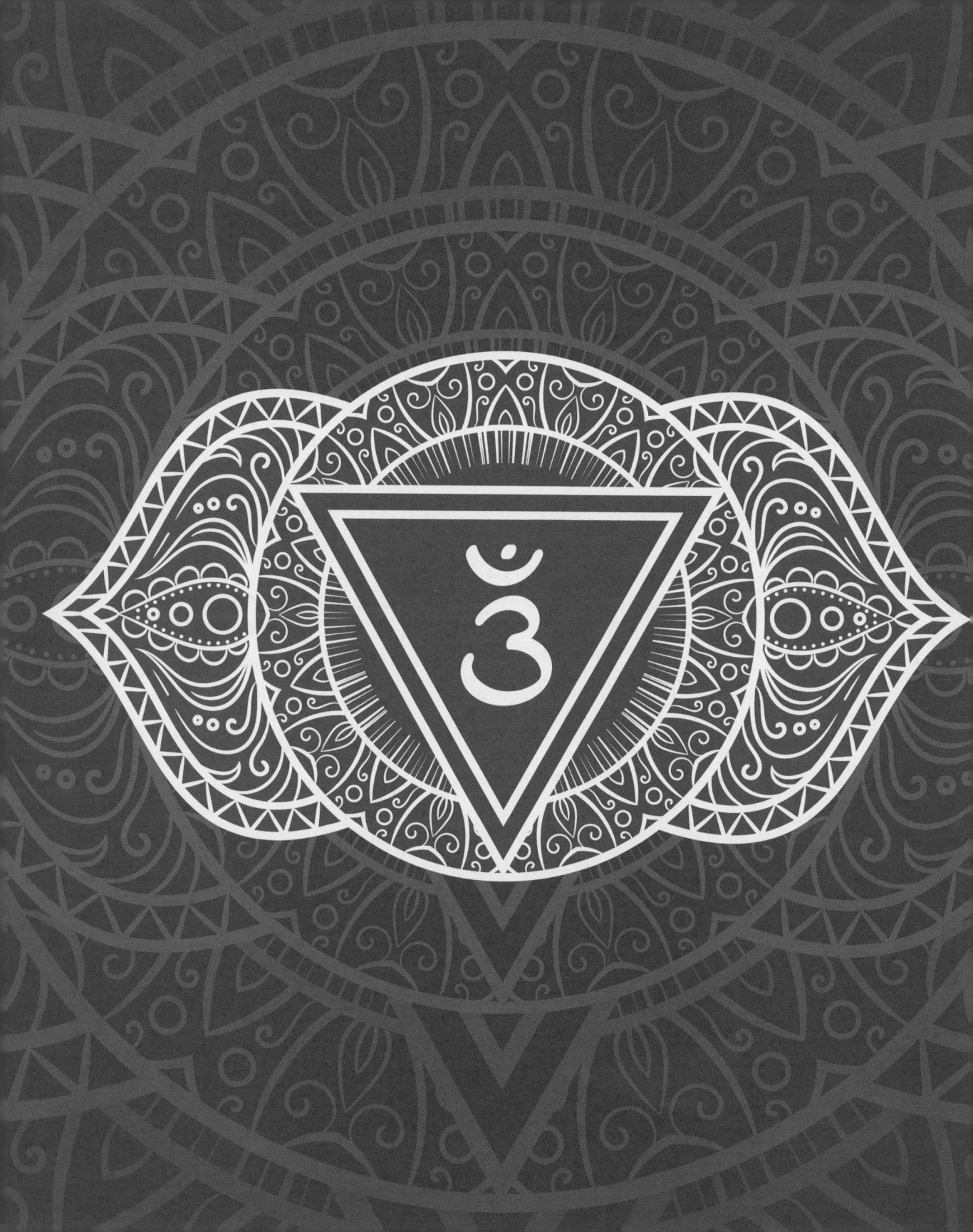

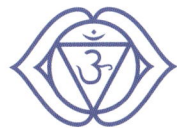

Third Eye Chakra

Ajna, the Sanskrit name for the third eye chakra, is generally translated as "to perceive" or "command." Thanks to its location at the center of the forehead, slightly above your eyebrows, it's sometimes referred to as the "brow chakra." This chakra is affiliated with our ability to see beyond what can be detected with the naked eye. It's spiritual and mystical and otherworldly, and it requires concentration and focus.

The third eye chakra relates to intuition, decision-making, and attention. It oversees the eyes, parts of the brain, and the pituitary and pineal glands. Sometimes simply rubbing the space between our brows can activate the third eye chakra, so accessible is this innate knowledge, if we're willing to listen.

To trust yourself, you have to hear yourself—and to hear yourself, you have to be calm, open, receptive, and focused. No distractions, whether from the external environment surrounding you or from your internal world, as when thoughts gambol and buck as chaotically as stormy waves. But you also need to be willing to accept whatever messages bubble up. Deepening our sight sometimes means seeing things we'd rather ignore or leave unacknowledged. So, it's important to have courage and to be brave. You have to believe in your inner wisdom and intuition, acknowledging their power to guide you.

WHY BALANCING YOUR THIRD EYE CHAKRA MATTERS

Like an animal pacing in its cage, sometimes our mind pounds well-worn paths. Instead of considering the evidence, we jump straight to conclusions, or we invent stories to justify our feelings. Balancing our third eye chakra keeps us from repetitive thinking. It helps us break familiar patterns and see things anew.

A balanced third eye chakra enables flashes of insight. You'll realize something you'd never thought of before, or see a situation with utter clarity. It's the cartoon lightbulb going off above your head, the perfect solution that comes to you in the shower, the penny dropping and happily rolling away. Of course, these realizations might not be easy. But living with discernment and understanding beats being mired in the same negative patterns of thought or behavior.

To understand the world, we need to utilize the intellectual and imaginative parts of our brain. Balancing the third eye chakra lets us employ both halves to their fullest capacity, rather than overrelying on one or the other. Our sight is clear, precisely because it's benefiting from thoughtfulness as well as a high emotional IQ.

What an Unbalanced Third Eye Chakra Feels Like

Unbalanced, our third eye chakra might cause us to become narrow-minded. We may fall prey to black-and-white thinking, have trouble differentiating between fiction and fact, or be reluctant to entertain multiple possibilities before making a decision. Rather than thinking and feeling in equal measure, we may tip too far to one side, neglecting the other.

An underactive third eye chakra inhibits our ability to think coherently about the future. Similarly, we might have trouble figuring out what we need to do in order to address whatever issues are preventing us from moving forward with the life we want to live. Yet, this stuckness can also occur with an overactive third eye chakra, with which we may have a hard time focusing. This inability to focus prevents us from identifying impediments and uncovering appropriate solutions.

A racing mind can be a sign of an overactive third eye chakra. You might have a hard time concentrating, because there's too much happening upstairs, or you might daydream excessively. Eventually, you might start to feel mentally foggy, as if thoughts were falling out of your head and into the ether, where they float away, never to be had again.

UNBALANCED THIRD EYE CHAKRA	
PHYSICAL AILMENTS	MENTAL AND EMOTIONAL AILMENTS
Headaches and migraines	Nightmares
Eye strain and other eye issues	Trouble concentrating
Insomnia	Brain fog
Dizziness	Excessive daydreaming
Sinus problems	Inability to make decisions

How to Balance Your Third Eye Chakra

Balancing your third eye chakra involves enhancing your focus, quieting your mind, and encouraging rest. When you're centered, you can act instead of react, decreasing your impulsivity and increasing your thoughtfulness. You'll let go of expectations around what should be. Your mind will be open, receptive, and clear.

Visualizations and Meditations

Spin the wheel. Envision an indigo wheel between your eyebrows, at the center of your forehead. Use your breath to make this wheel spin, or pace your breaths to its movement. As you watch the wheel turn, notice any sensations. Let yourself feel focused, untroubled, composed, and receptive.

Meditate on the color indigo. Picture a bunch of purple grapes or the night sky. Visualizing joyful bluish-purple things—like the ocean, a new pair of dark-wash jeans, or ripe eggplants—can help you unlock your third eye chakra. Wearing an item of indigo clothing can help, too, as can wearing your chakra bracelet.

THE SEVEN MAJOR CHAKRAS | *THIRD EYE CHAKRA*

Employ the 5-4-3-2-1 technique. If your mind is racing, you can't focus. If you can't focus, you can't intuit or perceive. This technique, sometimes referred to as the "five senses grounding," helps harness an overactive mind and returns it to the present from wherever your mind has sprinted off to. Take a deep breath. When you're ready, focus on your immediate surroundings and name:

- 5 things you can see
- 4 things you can touch
- 3 things you can hear
- 2 things you can smell
- 1 thing you can taste

The 5-4-3-2-1 technique reduces anxiety. Being in a tranquil state will help you access your third eye chakra and figure out what you need to do next (maybe nothing).

Do a focused meditation. This simple meditation encourages you to concentrate your awareness on a specific thing, such as a part of the body or object. Begin by getting comfortable and relaxing your breathing, then concentrate on whatever you've selected. That's it. If your mind wanders, guide it back. During a focused meditation, your goal is to acknowledge whatever comes up (like feelings of discomfort) without getting further agitated. You'll learn to cope with distractions and strengthen your powers of concentration, fundamental skills for your third eye chakra.

THE SEVEN MAJOR CHAKRAS | THIRD EYE CHAKRA

Color
Indigo

Element
Light

Sense
Sight

Crystals
Azurite, black obsidian, diamond, kyanite, sapphire

Essential Oils
Clary sage, patchouli, rosemary, sweet almond, vetiver

Food

Foods for your third eye chakra also benefit the brain, among them dark chocolate, oily fish like salmon and tuna, eggs, avocados, olive oil, and other healthy unsaturated fats, cruciferous vegetables such as cabbage and cauliflower, and seeds and nuts. Be careful with caffeine, though, which can kick the mind into overdrive.

Herbs and Spices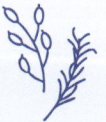

Chile, curry, ginseng, holy basil, mugwort

Yoga Poses and Stretches

Child's pose, dolphin pose, eagle pose, humble warrior, puppy pose

Breathwork
COHERENT BREATHING

Many cultures and religions practice some form of deep or coherent breathing, in which you slow your breathing to the rate of around five inhales and exhales per minute. This type of breathing can be done while sitting, standing, or lying down.

1. Lie flat, sit comfortably, or stand up straight.
2. Move your shoulders away from your ears. Relax.
3. Inhale for five counts.
4. Exhale for five counts.
5. Repeat this cycle of slow inhales and exhales for a full minute.
6. Resume breathing normally.

4-7-8 BREATHING

Like box breath (see page 60), 4-7-8 breathing involves timing your breath, in this case, four counts for the inhale and eight counts for the exhale with a seven-count pause in between. This breathwork has especially big benefits pre-sleep, as it lowers your heart rate and relaxes you.

1. Lie flat, sit comfortably, or stand up straight.
2. Move your shoulders away from your ears. Relax.
3. Inhale for four counts.
4. Hold for seven counts.
5. Exhale for eight counts.
6. Repeat for three or four more cycles.
7. Resume breathing normally.

Mantra Chant Sound

Om (pronounced *auuummm*)

Affirmations

I am wise and open to learning.
I trust my intuition.
My intuition leads me to wisdom.
I know what is best for me.
What I choose will be the right choice for me.

Flowers and Plants

Calathea, crocus, jade plant, lilac, spider plant

Acts of Service

Deep clean. Studies have found a connection between a messy environment and feelings of stress. Deep cleaning a loved one's space will not only increase their well-being (they'll be more relaxed!), but will also help improve your concentration. Here's how: Commit to immersing yourself. Rather than blasting a podcast or music as you scrub, be alone with your thoughts. Give yourself over to the task, then encourage your mind to roam. You may find yourself instinctively mulling over an issue or problem, and you may uncover clarity as you clean.

Be a sounding board. Helping someone with a tough decision can be an act of immense compassion and care. It requires listening without judgment, asking thoughtful questions, and giving worthwhile advice. Being a sounding board doesn't involve telling someone what you would do or critiquing someone's choices. Instead, the kind of valued counsel that will tune up your third eye chakra involves being open, kind, and empathetic. Deploying those characteristics for others will help us deploy them on ourselves when we're confronted with our own hard choice.

Everyday Activities to Activate Your Third Eye Chakra

Play board games. In recent years, board games have boomed. Nowadays, there are games about raising foxes, taking trains, settling imaginary lands, and everything in between. Whatever you're into, there's a board game that will enable you to spend quality time with friends or family, increase brain function, enhance dexterity, and otherwise add joy to your life (a boost for your sacral chakra, too). Regardless of whether you're playing to win, board games require you to shut out whatever else is going on and focus on what's in front of you—excellent training for your third eye chakra.

Time block. Also called "monotasking," time blocking involves setting aside a certain amount of time for a single task or focused work. For example, rather than checking your email every time you hear a ping, you might dedicate 30 minutes in the morning to responding to email and, again, in the afternoon. While many of us pride ourselves on our ability to multitask, research shows that multitasking leads to more distraction, more frustration, less focus, and, ultimately, less productivity.

Self-Care Rituals for Your Third Eye Chakra

Take good breaks. Resting is hard, especially when a deadline looms or you're in the middle of something. Yet, without rest, our brain and body begin to fatigue, causing us to be less productive in the long run. The best breaks get us away from whatever we're doing, letting us shift gears for a while. Go outside, have a healthy snack, or shut your eyes.

Unplug. Even if you're not always online, you probably receive hundreds of notifications per day. Researchers have found that it takes more than 20 minutes, on average, to get one's focus back after an interruption. Consider a social detox—even a short period away from screens can tamp down stress. Can't unplug? At the very least, aid your third eye chakra by reducing the number of notifications you receive each day.

Practice good sleep hygiene. Sleep matters, and yet most of us don't get enough. Increase your chances of getting a good night's sleep by improving your sleep environment and developing good sleep habits, also known as "sleep hygiene." Among the basics are avoiding screens for at least 30 minutes before bed, going to bed at a consistent time every day, keeping your room cool, and limiting bedroom activities to sleep and sex. Your entire chakra system will appreciate a well-rested you.

Journal Prompts

- *Write about a time when your intuition served you.*
- *What was the hardest decision you ever had to make? If you could go back, would you make the same decision?*
- *Does relaxing come easy to you? Why or why not?*
- *Who is the wisest person in your life?*
- *Which mindfulness practice has been most beneficial to you? How has it helped or changed you?*
- *Why does balancing your third eye chakra matter to you at this moment?*

THE SEVEN MAJOR CHAKRAS | THIRD EYE CHAKRA

THIRD EYE CHAKRA AT A GLANCE	
SANSKRIT NAME	Ajna (ag-nya)
SYMBOL	Lotus flower with two petals
LOCATION	Center of the forehead, slightly above the eyebrows
THIS CHAKRA IS CONNECTED TO	Imagination, intuition, perception, visualization
COLOR	Indigo
CRYSTALS	Azurite, black obsidian, diamond, kyanite, sapphire
ELEMENT	Light
MANTRA	Om
"I FEEL" AFFIRMATION	I feel wise
ANIMAL	Hawk
BENEFITS OF BALANCING THIS CHAKRA	Awareness, clarity, confident decision making, inner wisdom, self-trust
WHEN UNBALANCED	Capriciousness, distraction, mental fogginess, self-doubt, trouble sleeping or relaxing

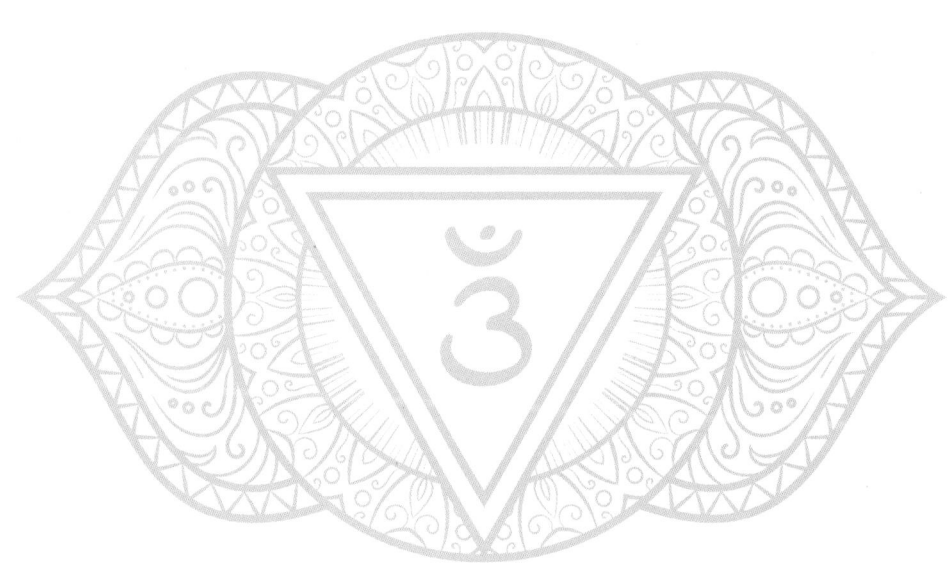

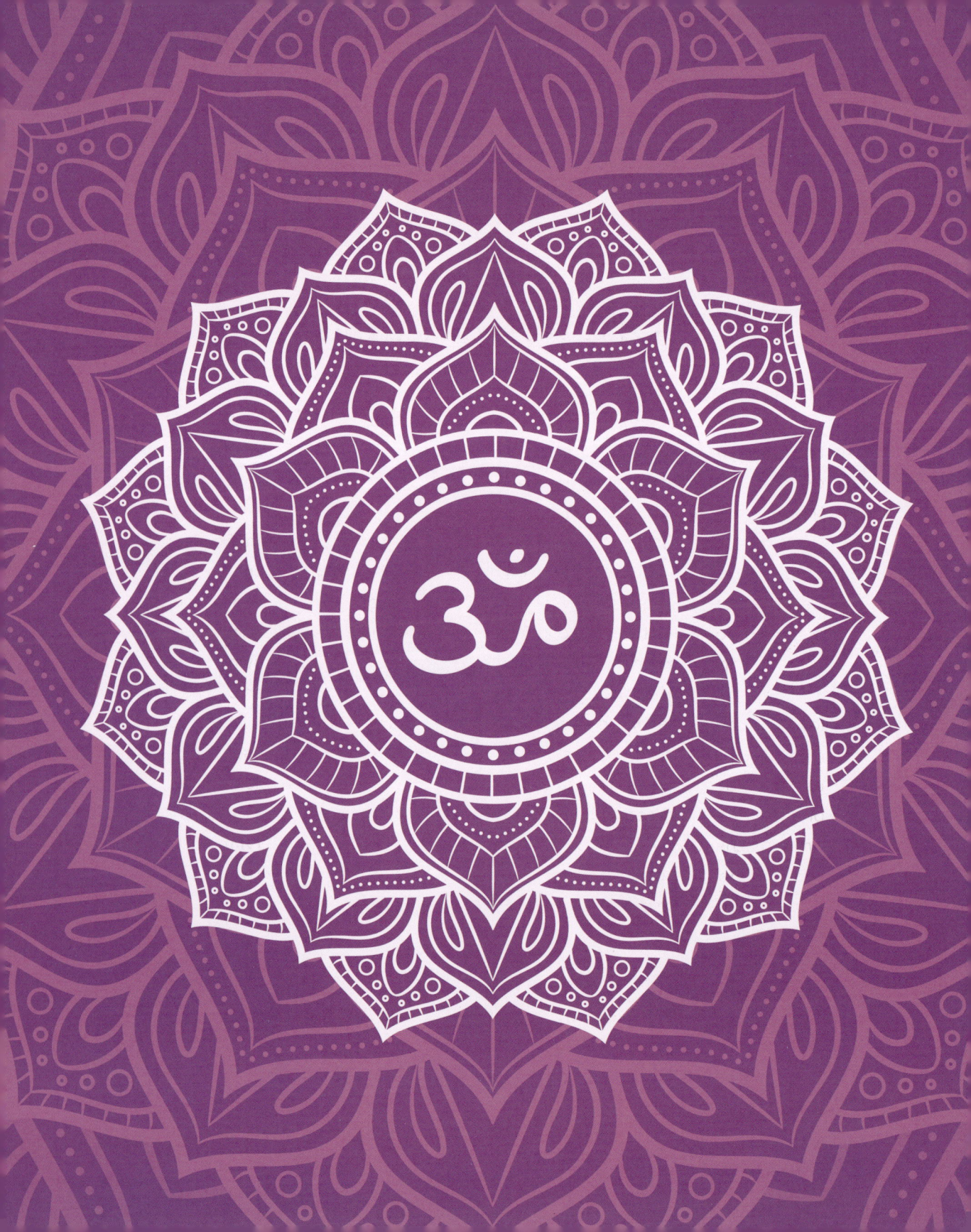

Crown Chakra

The crown chakra is the last of the seven major chakras. Balanced, our spiritual and physical sides co-exist in harmony. Unbalanced, this chakra can throw off our other major chakras, leading to a slew of ill effects, including depression, disconnection, low self-esteem, and stagnation. It's located at the top of the head, or crown.

When people speak about the crown chakra, they often talk, in the same breath, about divinity and spirituality. Through the crown chakra, we can become part of or deepen our connection to things that are greater than ourselves. For some, there's a comforting sense of smallness within a vastness, or a higher purpose operating within us that's accessible via the crown chakra.

"Higher power" may refer to the divine, but it might also mean universal love. For some, the crown chakra primarily brings up feelings of community and humanitarianism. In Sanskrit, the name for the crown chakra, *sahasrara*, means "thousand-petaled lotus." Each of us is an amazingly complex universe of thinking, feeling, sensing, and imagining, a world onto ourselves that orbits around other unique worlds full of the same potential and deserving of the same respect. Imagine the night sky brilliantly illuminated with starlight beaming in infinite directions.

WHY BALANCING YOUR CROWN CHAKRA MATTERS

Simply put, a balanced crown chakra helps you be the best version of yourself. You trust yourself, you believe in yourself, and you have faith in yourself. Armed with this self-assuredness, you're more empathetic and understanding toward others. You know that you have abundant gifts worth giving and sharing.

Because you're contently walking your own path, you're less concerned about what other people are doing, or not doing.

Balanced, the crown chakra enables you to feel as if you are exactly where you need to be. You are yourself, but also connected to something greater than yourself. You're energized by, and excited about, your purpose—not obnoxiously, arrogantly, or at the expense of anyone else, of course. Rather, you have a sense of where, how, and why you fit into the world. Some people refer to this feeling as "enlightenment." It's a harmonious balance between the spiritual and the physical.

In addition, a balanced crown chakra helps us let go of what no longer serves us. Shedding emotional baggage and laying down mental burdens, we begin to live with optimism, positivity, and grace. We're easy with others because we're easy in ourselves, and we're able to focus on what truly matters to us.

What an Unbalanced Crown Chakra Feels Like

When the crown chakra is unbalanced, we often struggle to think straight. We might feel overloaded with information, or we might feel chronically under-informed and three steps behind. A heavy, muddy brain can cause apathy and fatalism. We lose our sense of purpose and drive to achieve our goals. Our desire to act consciously and with verve goes away, replaced with an attitude of "So what?" and "What difference does it make?"

An underactive crown chakra walls us off. Closed-minded, we become dismissive of spiritual practices. Our minds narrow as our sense of connection withers. Because we are consumed by cynicism and afflicted with pessimism, the world becomes a dark place. Since the crown chakra impacts the other chakras, its imbalance causes other imbalances, a perilous cycle.

On the other end of the extreme, an overactive crown chakra frequently leads to rigidity and dogmatism. Our path becomes the only path, our beliefs the "correct" beliefs. Being too focused on otherworldly matters can cause quotidian matters to suffer, from neglecting relationships to forgetting about the business of everyday life.

UNBALANCED CROWN CHAKRA	
PHYSICAL AILMENTS	MENTAL AND EMOTIONAL AILMENTS
Headaches and migraines	Dogmatism
Sensitivity to sound and light	Pessimism
Hair loss	Obsessiveness
Sleep issues	Cynicism
Poor coordination and balance	Lack of direction

How to Balance Your Crown Chakra

Balancing the crown chakra requires letting go of our individual wants and needs (aka our ego), and turning our attention beyond ourselves. As such, the most impactful activities enable us to feel a part of something greater, such as a spiritual network or community, and they engender a sense of optimism about the future.

Visualizations and Meditations

Spin the wheel. Envision a violet or white wheel at the center of your chest (choose the color that speaks to you in the moment). Use your breath to make this wheel spin, or pace your breaths to its movement. As you watch the wheel turn, notice any sensations. Let yourself feel connected to the universe, full of the divine, or like the best possible version of yourself, ready to fulfill your life's purpose.

THE SEVEN MAJOR CHAKRAS | CROWN CHAKRA

Meditate on the color violet or white. Picture a perfectly made all-white bed or field of recently fallen snow. Visualizing joyful violet or white things—like clouds, swans, pearls, lambs, rows of blooming lavender or violets—can help you unlock your crown chakra. Wearing an item of violet or white clothing can help, too, as can wearing your chakra bracelet.

Visualize a light-filled lotus. Close your eyes and imagine a lotus flower floating above your head. As this flower opens, imagine its petals softly pouring light atop your head. Let this light spill down and onto your body. You may also chant "om" during this visualization. The crown chakra is connected to light—some people even see it as a halo.

Try the sahasrara mudra. Touch the tips of your thumbs and index fingers together to make a pyramid (the rest of your fingers should be spread out straight). Raise this mudra, or hand gesture, about 6 inches (15 cm) above the top of your head. Close your eyes and be silent, or chant *om*. Hold this position for 1–5 minutes.

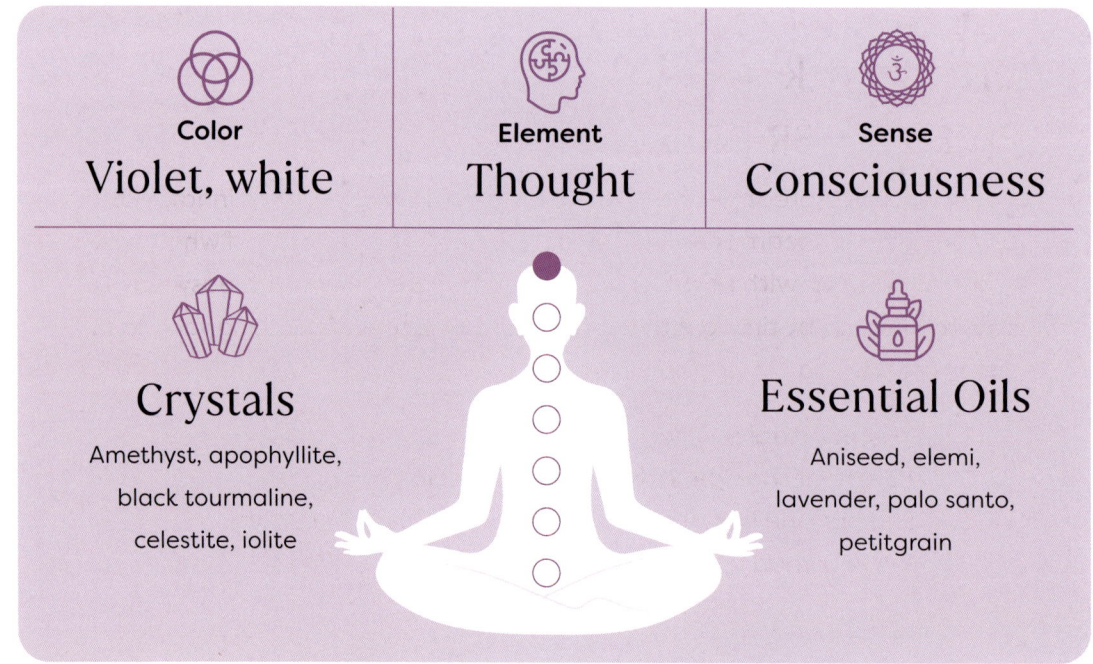

Color
Violet, white

Element
Thought

Sense
Consciousness

Crystals
Amethyst, apophyllite, black tourmaline, celestite, iolite

Essential Oils
Aniseed, elemi, lavender, palo santo, petitgrain

Food

Many religions and cultures use fasting as a mechanism for accessing the divine, increasing discipline, and aiding prayer. For these reasons, fasting is often recommended as an aid to opening the crown chakra. You could also eat white foods, like cauliflower, coconut, and garlic. Above all, remember to honor your food, including being grateful to those who helped grow or prepare it.

Herbs and Spices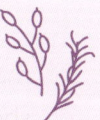

Ginkgo biloba, gotu kola, lemon balm, passionflower, St. John's wort

Yoga Poses and Stretches

Corpse pose, extended side angle, headstand, lotus or half-lotus pose, rabbit pose

Breathwork

FIVE-FINGER BREATHING

Counting one's breath—and aiming for a certain number of inhales and exhales—can sometimes lead to anxiety, exactly the opposite of what we're trying to achieve with breathwork. Five-finger breathing is an easy way to slow your breath by timing it to the physical movement of touching your hand. Instant relaxation.

1. Sit comfortably or stand up straight.
2. Move your shoulders away from your ears. Relax.
3. Hold out one hand, palm facing away from you or down. Gently spread your fingers.

4. Begin at the base of the thumb, where your hand meets your wrist, and use your pointer finger on the opposite hand to trace your open hand. Inhale as you go up each finger and exhale as you go down. Go as slowly as feels comfortable to you. Concentrate on the sensation of your finger sliding up and down your open hand, timing your inhales and exhales to the movement.
5. When you reach your pinkie, reverse the tracing, slowly re-tracing your fingers until you reach your thumb. Switch hands.
6. Repeat for a few cycles of breath.
7. Resume breathing normally.

SITALI BREATH

Sitali breath helps cool the body—when we're hot, we have a much harder time regulating our emotions. We're agitated, uncomfortable, and unable to concentrate. In this breathwork, you inhale through a rolled tongue and exhale through the nose. If rolling your tongue isn't available to you, purse your lips to inhale.

1. Sit comfortably or stand up straight.
2. Move your shoulders away from your ears. Relax.
3. Roll your tongue, as if the two sides could touch, to make a tube or taco shape, then extend your rolled tongue through your softly opened mouth as far as feels comfortable.
4. Inhale through the mouth. Feel the cool breath slide along your tongue.
5. Close your mouth and exhale through your nose.
6. Repeat this cycle at least five times.
7. Resume breathing normally.

Mantra Chant Sound ॐ

Om (pronounced *auuummm*)

Affirmations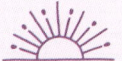

I am my best self, living my best life.
I inhale, then exhale what doesn't serve me.
The divine moves within me.
I am connected to the universe and all that dwells within it.
I accept myself, and I love myself.

Flowers and Plants

Echeveria,
lily of the valley,
lucky bamboo,
peace lily, snowdrop

Acts of Service

Volunteer for a cause you care about. Giving back activates what's known as a "helper's high." As we donate our time, talents, or resources, our brain releases endorphins, which, in turn, lead to positive emotions. Focusing on others takes the focus off ourselves. In addition, volunteering makes us feel connected to a broader community—we're working with like-minded individuals to contribute to the greater good.

Participate in a citizen science project. Sometimes called "participatory projects," these activities offer opportunities for ordinary people to contribute to meaningful scientific endeavors—no degree or experience is required. In some cases, you don't even need to leave your house. Being part of a project, such as searching for clouds on Mars or tracking butterflies in your neighborhood, creates a sense of connectedness and activates a sense of purpose. This work matters, as do our contributions.

Learn more about someone's spirituality. With an open mind and generous spirit, ask a friend to share their spiritual practice with you. Attend a service, or celebrate a holiday like Diwali. Participating in someone else's religious traditions not only broadens your mind and deepens your knowledge of the world, but it also reminds you that there are multiple means of accessing the divine.

Everyday Activities to Activate Your Crown Chakra

Take an awe walk. Awe connects us to the world by showing us something surprising or helping us see familiar things in exciting, new ways. It's easy to feel awed by an incredible natural wonder like the Grand Canyon, of course. But we can tap in to awe just by paying attention to what's around us, such as noticing wind moving through leaves on our morning commute.

Host a gathering. Feeling lonely has been shown to increase one's risk for all kinds of health problems and can lead to premature death. Combat social isolation by throwing a party—organize a board game night (which also benefits your third eye chakra!), or hold a picnic for parents and kids at a local park. The point is to convene a small crowd for some fun.

Make eye contact. The word *phubbing* might be fun to say, but it connotes the very real, and very sad, act of snubbing people in favor of looking at your phone. But we ignore people in other ways, too, such as when we keep our earbuds in during conversations or neglect to say "hello" or "thank you." We can increase our sense of connection by engaging with people around us, starting with eye contact.

Self-Care Rituals for Your Crown Chakra

Cultivate small joys. Life is hard—no news there—and we humans are hardwired to dwell on the negative, thanks to evolution: Ancestors who looked out for danger stayed alive. Combat the so-called negativity bias by seeking ways to cultivate joy in your life. Keep fresh flowers on your desk, wear a blazer for no reason, listen to a child tell jokes. Life is hard, sure, but it's in our power to make it a little less hard.

Make your own mandala. In Buddhism and Hinduism, the mandala often symbolizes the universe. Make your own by placing rocks, flower petals, and twigs in a circular pattern; drawing a mandala in your journal; or weaving yarn around sticks. Set aside expectations and concentrate on the act of creating. Let the creative act be the goal, thereby benefiting both your crown and sacral chakras.

Try a new spiritual practice. If you don't currently meditate, start. If you've never used crystals or essential oils, give them a try. Visit a religious site or museum—you don't need to be a believer to be moved by religious architecture, artifacts, or practices. Set aside your judgments and expectations about what you should think or how you should feel. Allow yourself to be open to new sensations.

Journal Prompts

- *Describe your ideal life, from what you're wearing to where you're living to who you're with and what you're doing.*
- *For what in your life are you most grateful?*
- *When or where do you feel most connected to something greater than yourself?*
- *What excites you about the future?*
- *When, where, and with whom do you feel like the best version of yourself?*
- *Why does balancing your crown chakra matter to you at this moment?*

CROWN CHAKRA AT A GLANCE	
SANSKRIT NAME	Sahasrara (sah-hass-rah-rah)
SYMBOL	Lotus flower with 1,000 petals
LOCATION	Top of head
THIS CHAKRA IS CONNECTED TO	The divine, enlightenment, spirituality, thinking and thought
COLOR	Violet, white
CRYSTALS	Amethyst, apophyllite, black tourmaline, celestite, iolite
ELEMENT	Thought
MANTRA	Om
"I FEEL" AFFIRMATION	I feel connected and whole
ANIMAL	Butterfly
BENEFITS OF BALANCING THIS CHAKRA	Feelings of interconnectedness, open-mindedness, optimism, serenity, sense of peace and well-being
WHEN UNBALANCED	Closed- or narrow-mindedness, dogmatism, lack of purpose, numbness, stubbornness

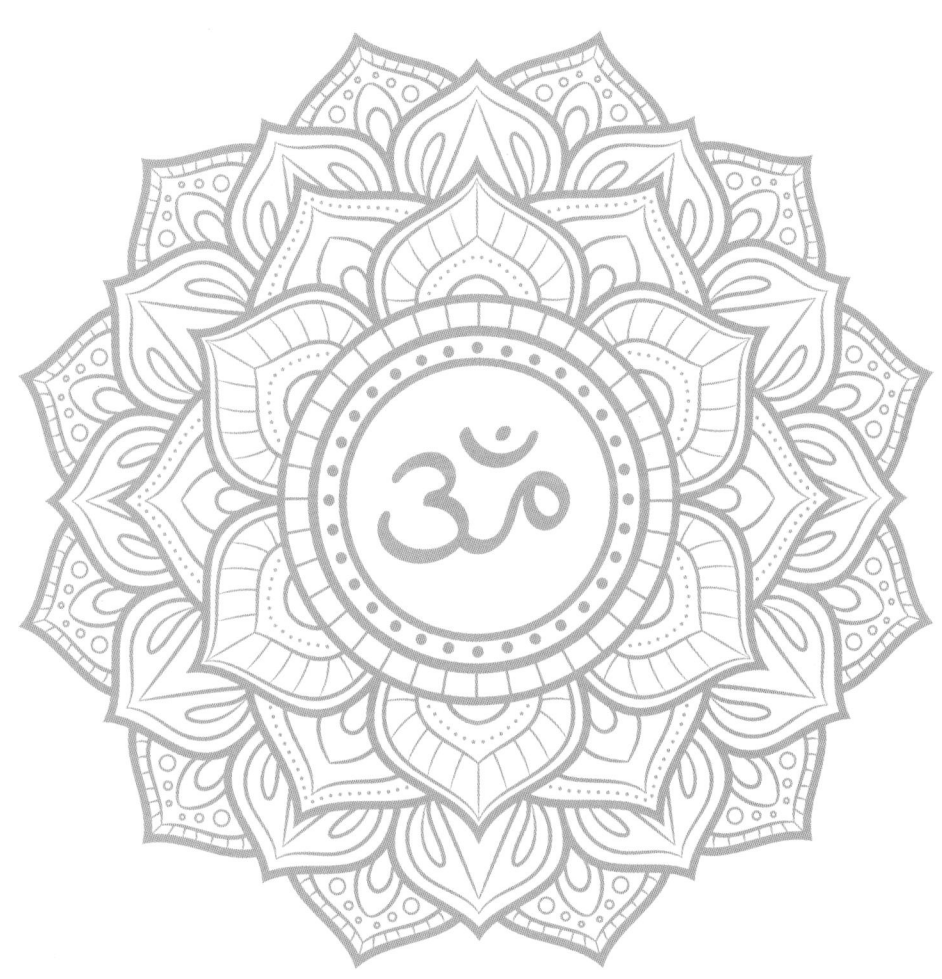

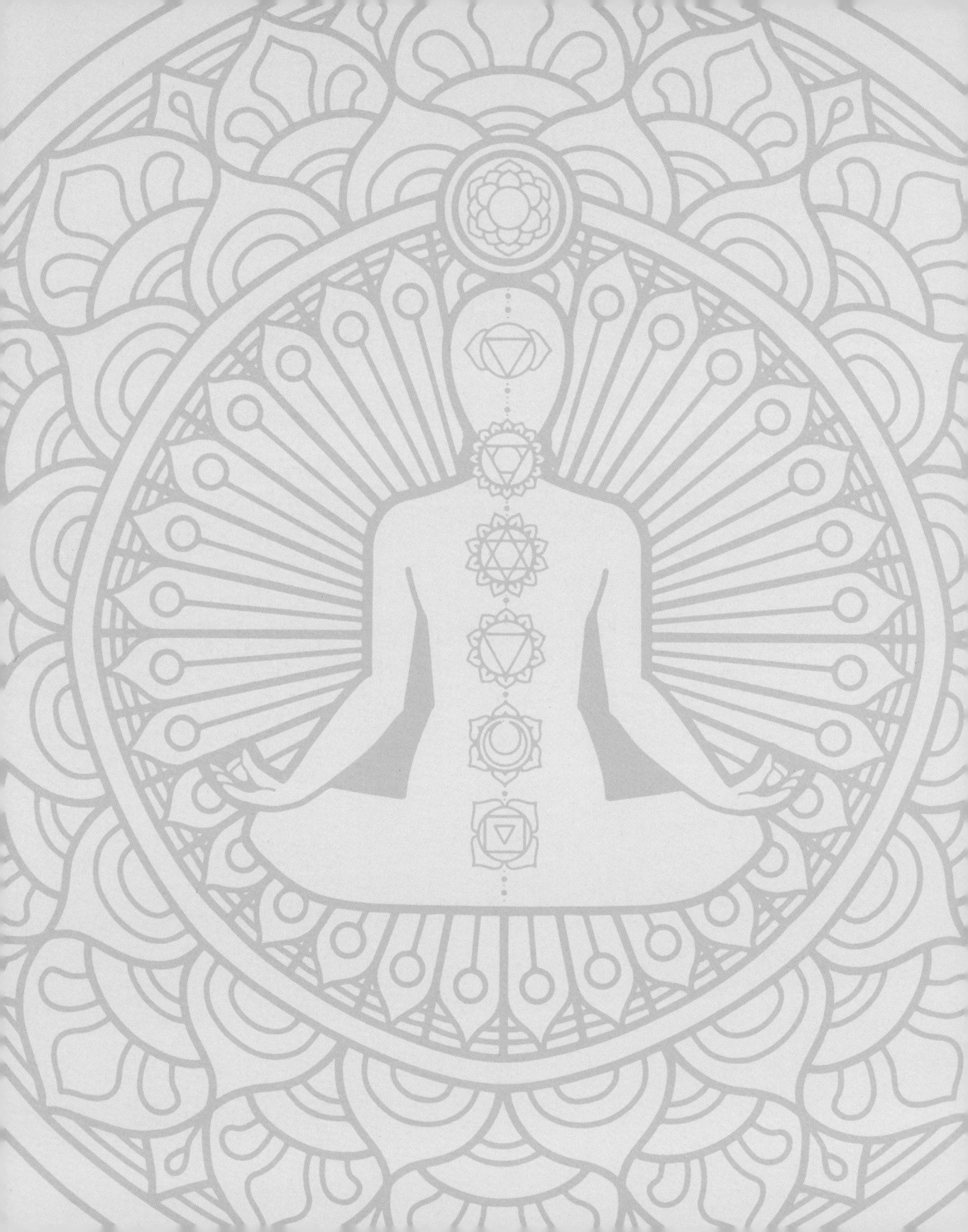

COMMON AILMENTS & AFFILIATED CHAKRAS

Refer to the following chart for a quick guide to common ailments and their affiliated major chakras. Then, turn to the relevant chakra chapter to explore strategies for relief, to remove blockages, and to help restore balance. Remember, though, the chakra system is interconnected so balancing one chakra can have a positive effect on the others.

COMMON AILMENTS & AFFILIATED CHAKRAS	
Anger	Heart Chakra, Solar Plexus Chakra
Anxiety	Heart Chakra, Root Chakra
Back pain	Heart Chakra, Root Chakra, Sacral Chakra
Cavities	Throat Chakra
Depression	Solar Plexus Chakra
Digestive issues	Root Chakra, Solar Plexus Chakra
Exhaustion	Crown Chakra, Sacral Chakra
Feeling meh	Root Chakra, Sacral Chakra

COMMON AILMENTS & AFFILIATED CHAKRAS

General Stiffness	Sacral Chakra
Indecisiveness	Third Eye Chakra
Insomnia/sleep disorders	Crown Chakra, Root Chakra, Third Eye Chakra
Jaw pain/grinding teeth	Throat Chakra
Knee pain	Root Chakra
Low self-esteem	Solar Plexus Chakra
Low sex drive	Sacral Chakra
Moodiness	Third Eye Chakra
Negativity/cynicism	Crown Chakra, Root Chakra
Poor posture (weak core)	Solar Plexus Chakra
Shoulder pain	Heart Chakra
Stiff neck	Throat Chakra
Stress	Root Chakra

STAY BALANCED

Chakras benefit from ongoing maintenance. Much the same as weeding a vegetable garden or taking your car for a tune-up, devoting a little time to regular chakra check-ins can ensure balance and prevent larger alignments later.

Revisit your journal. Re-read past entries to notice growth and change. You can also revisit prompts that speak to you, especially those related to why balancing a certain chakra matters to you at a given moment.

Take a crystal bath. One option for a crystal bath is to place a crystal on your body atop its corresponding chakra. You could also lie on a massage table with the crystals lined up beneath you, along your spine. Do one or more chakra visualizations as you bathe this way. Coupling breathwork with crystals can be deliciously impactful as well.

Develop a meditation practice. Promising research has shown that meditation offers a number of benefits, including better sleep, relaxation, and weight control along with positively impacting your chakras. Aim for at least 5 minutes per day, working up to a length of time that feels right to you (experts recommend 5–45 minutes per day). Above all, be consistent—meditating daily is more important than the length of time.

Eat a big salad. A salad full of colorful fruits and vegetables will not only make your body happy, but will also help your chakras. Aim for all the colors of the chakras, from red (root) to green (heart) to indigo (third eye). Don't forget herbs and spices, too.

Wear your bracelet. Since seeing or wearing a particular color can benefit its chakra, wearing your chakra bracelet can benefit the entire chakra system. Additionally, your chakra healing bracelet serves as a reminder to use your chakra cards, refer to your chart, thumb through this book, and otherwise tune in to your chakras.

Practice yoga regularly. Many people first learn about chakras through yoga, and moving through yoga's asanas (poses) is an excellent way to balance your system.

How to Balance Multiple Chakras at Once

If you're just starting your energy work, balancing a single chakra at a time might be easiest so you can really focus on it. In time, however, you may wish to balance multiple chakras at once. You can do so by combining a series of yoga poses into a routine. Another option is a full-body visualization in which you begin at the root chakra and move your way slowly and carefully up the body to the crown chakra (see pages 19–20 for guidance). I also recommend having a clear quartz on hand as this crystal is thought to help all chakras, and utilizing lavender oil as aromatherapy. Last but not least, wearing your chakra bracelet can benefit and align your entire chakra system.

Because the chakra system is interconnected, a great benefit of focusing on one chakra is its potential to aid another. For example, if you align your throat chakra, you feel more fully yourself, able to speak your truth and live authentically. This, in turn, helps your sacral chakra, as you'll feel more joyful and open to pleasure—and vice versa.

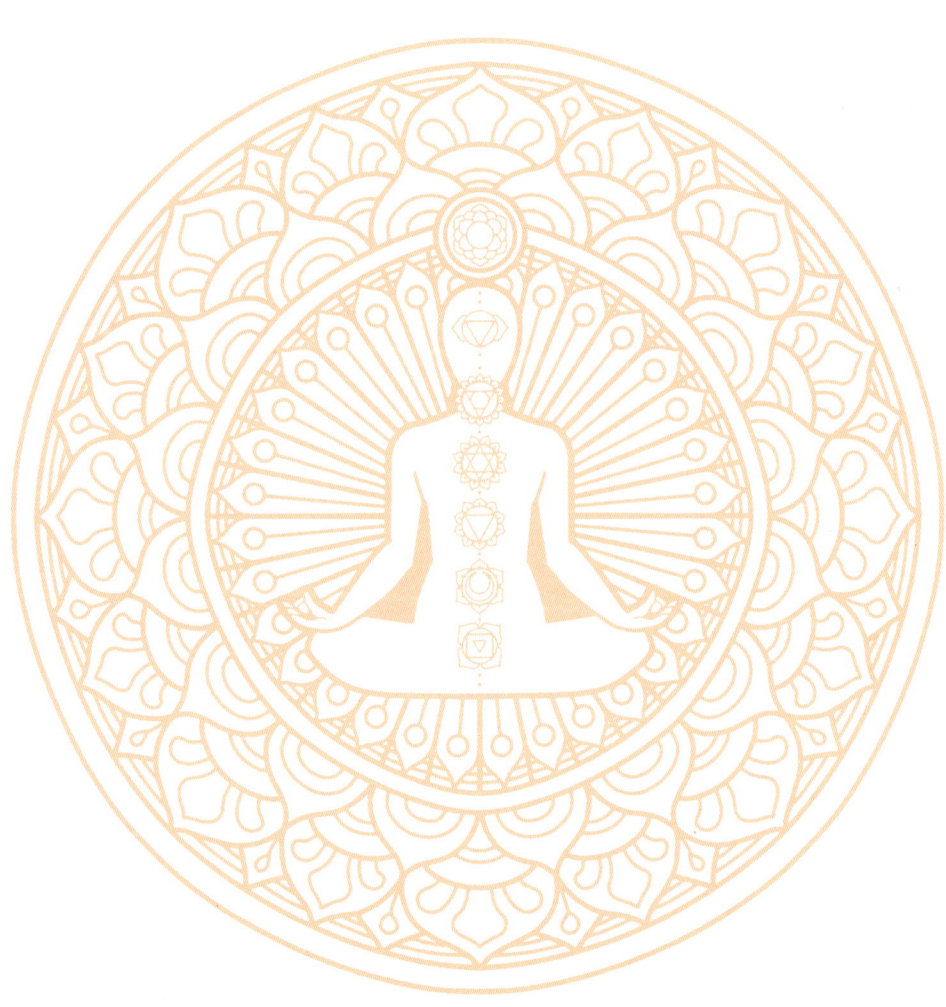

FINAL THOUGHTS

For some people, understanding the chakra system will complement a preexisting wellness practice, perhaps adding nuance to a yoga practice or ongoing breathwork. For others, understanding chakras will lead to further spiritual explorations. No matter where you are, I wish you well-being and peace on your journey. May you be the self you wish to be.

Our world holds much uncertainty. Yet we can say, with certainty, that who we are and how we act matter—a great deal, in fact. Understanding chakras helps us understand ourselves, including what we need in our lives as well as how we respond to the blessings and challenges that come our way. Working on improving ourselves has the potential to benefit not only us as individuals but also all with whom we come into contact, causing wonderful ripples that extend far, far beyond wherever and whoever we are.

ABOUT THE AUTHOR

Jessica Allen writes books about axolotls, numbers, astrology, poetry, and other interesting things. Her articles, reviews, and essays have been published in many places, including *The Boston Globe*, CNN, *The Independent*, McSweeney's, Mental Floss, The Onion's A.V. Club, *The Washington Post*, and *Writer's Digest*. She balances her chakras from her home in New York City, which she shares with her husband and their son.

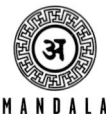

MANDALA

An Imprint of MandalaEarth
PO Box 3088
San Rafael, CA 94912
www.MandalaEarth.com

Publisher Raoul Goff
Associate Publisher Roger Shaw
Assistant Editor Amanda Nelson
Managing Editor Michelle Hope
Creative Director Ashley Quackenbush
Senior Designer Stephanie Odeh
VP Manufacturing Alix Nicholaeff
Production Manager Tiffani Patterson
Strategic Production Planner Lina s Palma-Temena

MandalaEarth would also like to thank Mary Cassells and Dominik Sklarzyk.

Text © 2025 Mandala Publishing

All rights reserved. No part of this book may be reproduced in any form without written permission from the publisher.

ISBN: 979-8-88762-175-3

This book is not intended as a substitute for the medical advice of physicians. The reader should regularly consult a physician in matters relating to their health, particularly with respect to any symptoms that may require diagnosis or medical attention.

Manufactured in China by Insight Editions
10 9 8 7 6 5 4 3 2 1

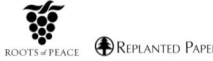

Insight Editions, in association with Roots of Peace, will plant two trees for each tree used in the manufacturing of this book. Roots of Peace is an internationally renowned humanitarian organization dedicated to eradicating land mines worldwide and converting war-torn lands into productive farms and wildlife habitats. Roots of Peace will plant two million fruit and nut trees in Afghanistan and provide farmers there with the skills and support necessary for sustainable land use.